Handbook of General Animal Nutrition

Udeybir Singh Chahal
B.V.Sc. & A.H., M.V.Sc., Ph.D.

P.S. Niranjan
B.Sc., B.V.Sc. & A.H., M.V.Sc. (*Gold Medalist*)

Sanjay Kumar
B.V.Sc. & A.H., M.V.Sc., Ph.D.

Department of Animal Nutrition
College of Veterinary Science & Animal Husbandry
Narendra Deva University of Agriculture & Technology
Kumarganj, Faizabad - 224 229 (U.P.), India

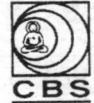

CBS Publishers & Distributors Pvt. Ltd.

New Delhi • Bengaluru • Chennai • Kochi • Mumbai • Pune
Hyderabad • Kolkata • Nagpur • Patna • Vijayawada

Handbook of General Animal Nutrition

ISBN: 978-81-239-2695-7

First CBS Reprint: 2015

Published by:
Satish Kumar Jain for CBS Publishers & Distributors Pvt. Ltd.,
4819/XI Prahlad Street, 24 Ansari Road, Daryaganj, New Delhi - 110002
delhi@cbspd.com, cbspubs@airtelmail.in • www.cbspd.com
Ph.: 23289259, 23266861, 23266867 • Fax: 011-23243014
Corporate Office: 204 FIE, Industrial Area, Patparganj, Delhi - 110 092
Ph: 49344934 • Fax: 011-49344935
E-mail: publishing@cbspd.com • publicity@cbspd.com

Branches:
• *Bengaluru:* 2975, 17th Cross, K.R. Road, Bansankari 2nd Stage,
  Bengaluru - 70 Ph: +91-80-26771678/79 • Fax: +91-80-26771680
  E-mail: cbsbng@gmail.com, bangalore@cbspd.com
• *Chennai:* No. 7, Subbaraya Street, Shenoy Nagar, Chennai - 600030
  Ph: +91-44-26681266, 26680620 • Fax: +91-44-42032115
  E-mail: chennai@cbspd.com
• *Kochi:* 36/14, Kalluvilakam, Lissie Hospital Road, Kochi - 682018
  Ph: +91-484-4059061-65 • Fax: +91-484-4059065
  E-mail: cochin@cbspd.com
• *Mumbai:* 83-C, Dr. E. Moses Road, Worli, Mumbai - 400018
  Ph: +91-9833017933, 022-24902340/41 • E-mail: mumbai@cbspd.com
• *Pune:* Bhuruk Prestige, Sr. No. 52/12/2+1+3/2,
  Narhe, Haveli (Near Katraj-Dehu Road Bypass), Pune - 411041
  Ph: +91-20-64704058/59, 32342277 • E-mail: pune@cbspd.com

Representatives:

• Hyderabad: 0-9885175004   • Kolkata: 0-9831437309, 0-9051152362
• Nagpur: 0-9021734563   • Patna: 0-9334159340
• Vijayawada: 0-9000660880

Printed at:
Neekunj Print Process, Delhi

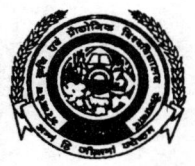

Narendra Deva University of
Agriculture & Technology
Kumarganj, Faizabad - 224 229
(U.P.), India

Dr. Basant Ram
Vice Chancellor

Foreword

I am very glad to know that *"Handbook of General Animal Nutrition"* authored by Dr. Udeybir S. Chahal, Dr. P.S. Niranjan and Dr. Sanjay Kumar is an epoch making effort put forth by faculty members of Animal Nutrition Department, Narendra Deva University of Agriculture & Technology, Kumarganj, Faizabad (UP) which extends the knowledge to students in excellent way. This is also the best procedure to demonstrate and discuss various theoretical aspect of animal nutrition as recommended by Veterinary Council of India. I am confident that this handbook will upgrade the knowledge and cater the basic need of undergraduate as well as post graduate students and other related persons in the field.

I congratulate the authors and International Book Distributing Company, Lucknow for this nice publication.

(Basant Ram)

Foreword

Preface

This book is prepared to cater the basic need of animal nutrition as a subject of B.V.Sc. & A.H. IInd year students and those who are preparing for JRF (Junior Research Fellowship) in animal sciences stream and also for civil services examination of different states. The animal nutrition Paper-I as per Veterinary Council of India (Minimum standards of Veterinary Education Degree) Regulation, 1993 includes two courses i.e. ANN- 211 (Principles of Animal Nutrition including avian, credit hr. 2+1) and ANN-212 (Evaluation of feed stuffs and feed technology, credit hr. 1+1) with equal weightage in internal assessment as well as external assessment of 50 percent each. The theory and practical portion has also equal weightage in internal and external examination with little variation at institutional level. This book is designed to cover all the material in a concise and course wise format. The objective and subjective questions at the end of each chapter and model test papers at the end of book will help the students for examination point of view. List of various books of Indian and Foreign authors which are thoroughly consulted to prepare this manuscript are also given at the end of this book. These suggested reference books are helpful for detailed study of each and every topic related to the field of animal nutrition.

The encouragement, guidance and foreword by our most reverend Dr. Basant Ram, Vice Chancellor, N.D.U.A. & T., Kumarganj, Faizabad (UP) is gratefully acknowledge.

At last authors thankfully acknowledge the help render by renowned personalities of animal nutrition, scientist, faculty members, colleagues, friends, family members, supporting staffs and all those whose designation are not mentioned here. Authors hope that this book achieves its objective and popularity among students, research scholars, teachers and all concerned persons.

Udeybir S. Chahal
P.S. Niranjan
Sanjay Kumar

ANN-211: Principles of Animal Nutrition (including Avian Nutrition) Cr. Hrs. 2+1=3

Theory: History of animal nutrition, importance of nutrients in animal health and production, composition of animal body and plants, comparison between plants and animals, biochemical basis of soil, plant and animals. Nutritional terms and their definitions. Nutrients and their metabolism, role and requirements of water. Carbohydrates – their digestion, absorption and metabolism in ruminants and non-ruminants. Proteins and amino acids, their digestion, absorption and metabolism. Use of NPN compound for ruminants and non-ruminants. Lipids and their utility. Mineral elements and their functions – major elements. Importance of trace elements in livestock health and production. Importance of vitamins, their deficiency symptoms, requirements of supplementation in feed. Feed additives in the rations of livestock and poultry; antibiotics and hormonal compounds and other growth stimulants; their uses and abuses.

Practical: General precautions while working in nutrition laboratories. Normal solution, equivalent weight, molar and normal solutions, titration, standard solution, titer, end point and indicators. Preparation of solutions of various strength of common acids, alkalies and alcohols for determination of proximate principles of feed. Preparation of common reagents and indicators. Preparation of samples for chemical analysis – herbage, faeces, silage. Processing and weighing of biological samples – weighing of sample for proximate analysis, general precautions in weighing samples. Proximate principles in feed – general views, main features of Weende's system of analysis, estimation of dry matter, total ash and acid insoluble ash in feed samples. Familiarization of various feed stuff, fodders and their selection.

Lecture schedule: Principles of Animal Nutrition (including Avian Nutrition)

Topics	No. of lectures
Introduction and history of animal nutrition	2
Importance of nutrients in animal health and production.	2
Composition of animal body and plants; soil, plant and animal relationship.	3
Nutritional terms and their definitions.	2
Role and requirements of water.	2
Digestion, absorption and metabolism of carbohydrates in non-ruminants.	3
Digestion, absorption and metabolism of carbohydrates in ruminants.	2
Digestion, absorption and metabolism of proteins in non-ruminants.	3
Digestion, absorption and metabolism of proteins in ruminants.	2
Use of NPN compound for ruminants and non-ruminants.	2
Digestion, absorption and metabolism of lipids in non-ruminants.	2
Digestion, absorption and metabolism of lipids in ruminants.	2
Importance of major and trace mineral elements in livestock health and production, deficiency symptoms and mineral content of various feeds.	5
Importance of vitamins, their deficiency symptoms, requirements of supplementation in feed.	5
Feed additives in the rations of livestock and poultry; antibiotics and hormonal compounds and other growth stimulants, their uses and abuses.	3

ANN: 212 (Evaluation of Feed Stuffs and Feed Technology) Cr. Hrs. 1+1=2

Theory: Common feeds and fodders, their classification, availability and importance for livestock and poultry production. Chemical composition and nutritive value of various feeds and fodders. Measures of food energy and their applications- gross energy, digestible energy, metabolisable energy, net energy, total digestible nutrients, starch equivalent, food units, physiological fuel value. Direct and indirect calorimetry, carbon and nitrogen balance studies. Protein evaluation of feeds – Measures of protein quality in ruminants and non-ruminants, biological value of protein, protein efficiency ratio, protein equivalent, digestible crude protein. Calorie protein ratio. Nutritive ratio. Various physical, chemical and biological methods of feed processing for improving the nutritive value of inferior quality roughages. Preparation, storage and conservation of livestock feed e.g. silage and hay making and their use in livestock feeding. Harmful natural constituents and common adulterants of feeds and fodders.

Practical: Determination of proximate principles of feed-estimation of crude protein, ether extract, crude fiber, nitrogen free extract, calcium and phosphorus in feed samples. Demonstration of detergent methods of forage analysis. Qualitative detection of undesirable constituents and common adulterants of feed. Demonstration of laboratory ensiling of green fodders. Feed mixing (selection of material for quality control, feed processing). Silage pit preparation.

Lecture schedule: Evaluation of Feed Stuffs and Feed Technology

Topic	No. of lectures
Common feeds and fodders, their classification, availability and importance for livestock and poultry production.	3
Chemical composition and nutritive value of various feeds and fodders.	2

Topic	No. of lectures
Measures of food energy and their applications- gross energy, digestible energy, metabolizable energy, net energy, total digestible nutrients, starch equivalent, physiological fuel value.	3
Direct and indirect calorimetry, carbon and nitrogen balance studies.	2
Protein evaluation of feeds – Measures of protein quality in ruminants and non-ruminants, biological value of protein, protein efficiency ratio, protein equivalent, digestible crude protein, calorie protein ratio and nutritive ratio	3
Various physical, chemical and biological methods of feed processing for improving the nutritive value of inferior quality roughages.	2
Preparation, storage and conservation of livestock feed e.g. silage and hay making and their use in livestock feeding	3
Harmful natural constituents and common adulterants of feed and fodders.	2

Contents

PART-I

Course No. ANN- 211 (Principles of Animal Nutrition (including Avian Nutrition))

Chapter 1

History of Animal Nutrition

Definition of Animal Nutrition:

Animal nutrition is made up of two words i.e. animal and nutrition. Dictionary means of animal is any living thing, other than a human being, that can feel and move or a creature with four legs, as distinct from a bird, a reptile, a fish or an insect. Examples are cattle, sheep, goat, horse, dogs and cat etc. In dictionary terms, nutrition is "The series of processes by which an organism takes in and assimilates food for promoting growth and replacing worn or injured tissues". Therefore, nutrition involves various chemical reactions and physiological processes, which transform foods into body tissues and activities. It involves the ingestion, digestion, and absorption of the various nutrients, their transport to all body cells, and the removal of unusable elements and waste products of metabolism. So, animal nutrition is the science of nourishment of animals.

History of Animal Nutrition:

Antoine Lavoisier (1743-1794) was the founder of the science of nutrition. He was the father of nutrition. He established the chemical basis of nutrition and stated that life is a chemical process. He introduced the balance and thermameter int nu.rition studies and designed a calorimeter with Laplace. At the beginning, it was believed that nutritive value of food resided in a single aliments. But in early nineteen century it was proved wrong. William Prout reported that nutrient constituent of animal body were provided by three principals i.e. saccharine (carbohydrate), oily (lipid) and albuminous (protein).

In mid 19th century Chosset observed that pigeons on low calcium diet had poor bone development. The importance of other minerals like chlorine, magnesium, sodium, potassium and sulphur were also known during this period.

In late 19th century Takaki observed that Beri-Beri disease can be prevented by dietary supplementation. All the vitamins were discovered during the period of 1910-1950.

Stephen M. Babcock (1843-1931) conducted first feeding experiment with single plants. All the grain and forage were from either corn or wheat plants. It stimulated the use of the purified diet method, which resulted in discovery of vitamins.

In 20th century various vitamins, minerals, amino acids, fatty acids and their role had been discovered. Various feeding standards indicating the requirements of various nutrients for various categories of livestock for different functions were established. Various non-conventional feeds were discovered as livestock feed. Various economical and balanced rations were prepared for different categories of livestock. So a lot of work has been done in 20th century. Even than, there is a great scope for further improvement and new research in the field of animal nutrition in 21st century. For which a lot of research work is on progress at various research centers and dept. of Animal Nutrition in various College of Veterinary Sciences & Animal Husbandry throughout the country and abroad, with a hope of further improvement and new research in the field of animal nutrition which will benefit the society in many ways and full fill the objective to provide all essential nutrients in adequate amount and in optimum proportions at least cost of feeding to the animals.

Relationship with other branches of sciences: Animal nutrition has a direct relationship with Physics, Chemistry, Biochemistry, Physiology, Genetics and Breeding, Anatomy and Histology, Biology, Mathematics and Microbiology without which complete study of animal nutrition is impossible. So relative study of other sciences are also necessary and helpful for the animal nutritionists.

Role of nutrition in animal production and health: The factors responsible for efficient animal production are:
1. Genetic potentiality of animal
2. Nutritional status of animal
3. Managemental factor

Nutrition plays an important role in the animal production and health by following ways:
1. It exploites the genetic potentiality of the animal. For example if a cow has capacity to produce 30 litre of milk per day (by its genetic make up) but it can not be possible if the cattle is under fed.
2. It makes the animal production cheap and economical. Because cost of feeding and feeds accounts for 70-80% of total animal production cost. So it is the major means by which production system can be made economical.
3. It also minimizes the competition between human and animal for food by introducing non-conventional feed ingredients for animal feeding.
4. It also manipulates feed ingredients for effective utilization of nutrients. In this way nutrition play an important role in animal production and health.

Milestones in the development of Animal Nutrition:

Sr. No.	Scientists	Contribution
1.	A Lavosier (1762)	Nature of respiration, calorimetery.
2.	William Prout (1834)	Nature of food
3.	Max Rubner (1908)	Energy metabolism
4.	G.J. Mulder (1838)	Gave the name protein
5.	J.B. F. Magendie (1783-1855)	Essentiality of food nitrogen

6.	Lawes and J.H. Gilbert (1855)	Slaughter experiment in farm animals
7.	W.O. Atwater (1892)	First human respiration calorimeter
8.	Oscar Kellner (1851-1911)	Starch equivalent system of energy evaluation
9.	H.P. Armsby (1851-1921)	Respiration calorimeter for farm animals
10.	Leonard A. Maynard (1942)	Chairman of the NRC committee on animal nutrition
11.	Max Kleiber (1893-1976)	Use of the weight to the 0.75 power instead of surface area for energy metabolism.
12.	E.J. Underwood (1905-1980)	Mineral nutrition in livestock
13.	A. Bhattacharya (1980)	Study of recycling poultry waste as feed stuffs.
14.	P.J. Van Soest (1960)	Fibre estimation in feed stuffs
15.	Henneberg and Stohman (1861)	Proximate analysis of feed stuffs
16.	Indian Veterinary Research Institute, Izatnagar, (1939)	Various research in animal nutrition
17.	National Dairy Research Institute, Karnal (1952)	Various research in animal nutrition
18.	K.C. Sen (1954)	Nutritive value of Indian cattle feeds and feeding of farm animals
19.	N.D. Kehar (1950)	Nutritive value of non-conventional feeds. Wet alkali treatment to straw
20.	S.K. Talapatra (1964)	Methods to estimate minerals in feeds and fodders

21.	Indian Council of Agricultural Research (1985)	Feeding standard for various categories of livestock.
22.	K. Pradhan	Chairman of Committee to develop ICAR feeding standard.
23.	NRC (National Research Council, USA)1942	Nutritient requirements for livestock
24.	ARC (Agriculture Research Council, U.K.) 1959	Nutritient requirements for livestock.
25.	Hungate (1966)	Rumen microbiology
26.	Casimir Funk (1912)	Gave term vitamine

Nutrition definitions and terms: There are various term and definitions used in animal nutrition which are described as:

Nutrition: Nutrition involves various chemical reactions and physiological processes, which transform foods into body tissues and activities.

Animal Nutrition: Science of nourishment of animals.

Nutrient: The chemical substances found in the feed materials are necessary for the maintenance, production and health of animals. The chief classes of nutrients include- 25 carbohydrates, 15 fatty acids, 20 amino acids, 15 essential and 10 probably essential minerals, 20 vitamins and water or any chemical compound having specific functions in the nutritive support of animal life.

Nutriment: Any thing that promotes growth or development.

Nutriture: Nutritional status.

Health: Health is the state of complete physical, mental and social well being and not merely the absence of disease or infirmity as defined by World Health Organization.

Nutritious: Substances that promote growth and participate in repairing tissues of the body.

7

Nutritionist: A specialist in the problems of nutrition.

Nourish: To feed an animal with substance necessary for life and growth.

Feed (Feed stuff): Food of animals comprising any naturally occurring ingredient or material fed to animals for the purpose of sustaining growth and development.

Diet: A regulated selection of a feed ingredient or mixture of ingredients including water, which is consumed by animals on a prescribed schedule.

Ingredients: Any of the feed items that a mixture is made of.

Additives: An ingredient or a combination of ingredients added to the basic feed mixture for specific purposes like to increase feed ingestion or to alter metabolism.

Ration: A fixed amount of feed for one animal, fed for a definite period, usually for a 24 hour period.

Balanced ration: The ration which provide an animal with the proper amount, proportion and variety of all the required nutrients to keep the animal in its form to perform best in respect of production and health.

Complete ration: A single feed mixture, which has all of the dietary essentials except water for a given class of livestock.

Purified diet: A mixture of the known essential dietary nutrients in a pure form that is fed to experimental animals in nutrition studies.

Fortify: Nutritionally, to add one or more nutrients to a feed.

Limiting amino acid: The essential amino acid of protein that shows the greatest percentage deficit in comparison with the amino acids contained in the same quantity of another protein selected as standard.

Bran: The pericarp or seed coat of grain removed during processing.

Groat: Grain from which hulls have been removed.

Zein: A protein of low biological value present in maize, deficient in lysine and tryptophane amino acid.

Fodder: Aerial parts with ears, with husks or heads.

Stover: Thick solid stem and aerial parts without ears, husks or heads while harvesting maize, jowar commonly the earheads is removed and the remaining dried portion can be classed as stovers i.e. jowar and maize stover.

Hull: Outer covering of beans, peas, cotton seeds.

Husk: Dry outer covering of grains i.e. rice husk, gram husk.

Shells: Hard outer covering of nuts e.g. groundnut shell.

Corn cobs: After removal of corn grains.

Hay: Hay is the product obtained by drying in the sun or in the shade, tender stemmed leafy plant material in such a way that they contain not more than 12-14 percent moisture.

Straw: Straw is the by-product of any cereal, millet or legume crop left over after harvesting, threshing and removal of the grains or pulses.

Bagasse: It is the fibrous material left over in the sugar factories after extraction of all the juice from sugar cane.

Gluten: When flour is washed to remove the starch, a tough viscid, nitrogenous substance remains. This is known as gluten.

Germ: It is the embryo of any seed.

Meal: Feed ingredients of which the particle size is larger than flour.

Shorts: A by-product of flour milling consisting of a mixture of small particles of bran and germ, the aleurone layer and coarse fibre.

Malt sprouts: The radical of the embryo of the grain

removed from sprouted and steamed whole grain. These are obtained as by-products of liquor processing.

Red dog: By product of milling spring wheat consists primarily of the aleurone with small amounts of flour and fine bran particles.

Alkaloids: Alkaloid constitutes a large number of the active principles of plants and all possess a powerful physiological action.

Anatoxin: A toxin rendered harmless by heat or chemical means but capable of stimulating the formation of antibodies.

Antizymotic: An agent, which inhibits fermentation.

Avitaminosis: A condition produced by a deficiency or lack of a vitamin in the food.

D-value: It is percentage of digestible organic matter in the dry matter of the feed. It describes the digestibility of animal feed.

In vitro: Literally "in glass" pertaining to biological experiments performed in test tubes or other laboratory vessels.

In vivo: Within the living organisms pertaining to the laboratory testing of agents within living organisms.

Effluent: Liquid waste from an abattoir or slurry.

Gavage: Feeding an animal by means of a stomach tube.

Feed Conversion efficiency (FCE): The gain in weight in Kg or lb, produced by one Kg or one lb of feed. It is reciprocal of the feed conversion ratio.

Feed conversion ratio (FCR): The amount of feed in Kg or lb necessary to produce one Kg or one lb of weight gain.

Calorie: A unit of measurement used for calculating the amount of energy produced by various foods. It is the amount of heat needed to raise the temperature of 1 gram of water by 1^0C (14.5^0C-15.5^0C).

Proteins: These are complex nitrogenous organic chemical compounds specially made up of C,H, O, S and a large but fairly constant amount of nitrogen.

Mineral or Ash or inorganic element: A substance is ashed to the extent that there is no black particle left, the remaining portion is called mineral or ash.

Non-protein Nitrogenous compounds (NPN): Certain substances that do not contain protein but are rich in nitrogen content e.g. Urea, amides and ammonium salt.

Forage/Roughage: Poor quality feeds containing lesser amount of total digestible nutrients (TDN) or more than 35 percent cell wall constituents and more than 18 percent of crude fibre (CF).

Concentrate: It contains little amount (less than 18 percent) of crude fibre and more than 60 percent total digestible nutrient.

Probiotics: Probiotics are viable defined microorganisms in sufficient numbers, which alter the microflora of the host intestine and by that exert beneficial health effects on the host.

Silo: A semi-air tight structure designed for use in production and storage of silage.

Q.1 Fill in the blanks:

1. A French chemist – – – – – is known as father of sciences of nutrition.

2. ICAR feeding standard was developed in – – – – – – year under the chairman ship of – – – – – – – – – –.

3. S.K. Talapatra developed methods to estimate – – – – – in feeds and fodder.

4. IVRI Izatnagar was established in year– – – – – – – – –.

5. NDRI Karnal was established in – – – – – – year.

6. Proximate analysis of feed stuffs was given by – – – – – – – – and – – – – – –.

7. The term protein was derived by – – – – – – – – – – – – – –.

8. William Prout (1834) explained the — — — — — — — — — — .

9. Study of recycling poultry waste as a feed stuff is given by — — — — — — — .

10. NRC, started publication of Nutrient requirement for live-stock in year — — whereas ARC start it in — — — — — — — — —-

11. Biological experiments performed in test tube is called — — — — — — — — — — .

12. An agent which inhibits fermentation is known as — — — — — — — — — — — — .

13. Embryo of any seed is called — — — — — — — — where as hard outer covering of nuts is called — — — — — — — — — — .

14. A fixed amount of feed for an animal fed for a 24 hour period is called — — — — .

15. A protein of low biological value present in *Zea maize* is referred as — — — — — — .

16. — — — — — — — — (1843-1931) conducted first feeding ex-periment with single plant.

Q.2 Write short notes on the following :

1. Mention the contribution of five scientists in the field of animal nutrition.

2. Name the three national institutes involved in research activities attires in the field of animal nutrition.

3. Mention the name of five books of animal nutrition with their author or authors including three Indian authors' books.

4. How nutrition play important role in animal production and health. ?

5. Mention any five researches, which proveu to be a mile-stone in the field of animal nutrition.

Chapter 2

The Composition and Comparison of Plants and Animal Body

The chemical composition of plant and animal represents all the physical and chemical basis of protoplasm of the living processes, which occur in it. The animal body derives all the nutrients for its physiological functions from the digestion of plant and plant products with limited amount of animal origin feeds such as fish meal and milk. So a brief consideration of the chemical composition of the animal in relation to the composition of its food is useful to give a general picture of the nutritional process. We must know the chemical composition of farm animals to understand their nutrient requirement and composition of plants because they furnish most of the food for livestock.

Chemical composition of plants and animals: Plants and animals tissues are made up of similar type of chemical substances but their relative amounts are variable. Plants are analysed by proximate method of analysis given by Henneberg and Stohmann (1861). Whereas, animal body was first analysed by Lawes and Gilbert (1858) by slaughter experiments. Most of the nutrients present in plants and animals are arranged in to six groups, which are water, protein, carbohydrate, fat, mineral and vitamin. Plants and their by-products show much larger differences in the chemical composition than the animals.

Plants synthesize complex materials from simple substances such as carbondioxide, water, nitrates and other mineral salts from the soil and energy trapped from the sun by the process of photosynthesis. The greater parts of the energy trapped as a chemical energy within the plant itself and the animals use this energy. Thus, plants store and animals dissipate energy. The approximate chemical compositions of some plants, animals and their by-products have been given in Table 2.1.

Table 2.1 Approximate percent chemical composition of some plants, animals and their by-products

	Water	Crude protein	Fat	Carbohydrates	Ash
Green plants					
Berseem	90.0	2.0	0.3	6.3	1.4
Cowpea	80.0	2.50	0.5	15.0	2.0
Maize	75.0	2.0	0.6	21.0	1.4
Pasture grass (Young leafy)	84.0	3.60	1.0	10.0	2.4
Cereal grains					
Wheat	13.0	12.0	2.0	71.2	1.7
Groundnut	6.0	27.0	45.0	20.0	2.0
Plant by- product					
Wheat straw	10.0	3.5	1.5	76.5	8.5
Paddy straw	10.0	3.5	1.5	70.5	14.5
Wheat bran	10.0	10.0	3.0	70.0	7.0
Rice bran	10.0	10.0	15.0	55.0	10.0
Animal					
New born calf	74.0	19.0	3.0	-	4.0
Dairy cow	57.0	17.0	21.6	-	5.0
Sheep	74.0	16.0	5.0	-	4.4
Pig	60.0	13.0	24.0	-	3.0
Hen	57.0	21.0	19.0	-	3.0
Animal by-product					
Blood	82.0	16.4	0.6	0.1	0.7
Muscles	72.0	21.4	4.5	0.6	1.5
Milk	87.0	3.5	4.0	4.7	0.8

Basis of expressing the chemical composition: The chemical composition of the feed stuffs can be expressed in two ways-

1. **On fresh basis (as such basis):** On as such basis means expressing the chemical composition of the feed as is fed to the animals. The advantage of this expression is that it helps in computation of ration.

2. **On dry matter basis:** Chemical composition of feed stuffs is expressed on dry matter basis. The advantage of dry matter basis is that various feed stuffs can be compared among themselves by bringing at same standard unit of measurements. The average chemical composition in round figures of the common Indian feed stuffs is given in Table-2.2.

Table 2.2 : Chemical composition of some common feed stuffs

Feed stuffs	DM	CP	EE	CF	NFE	Ash	Ca	P
Straw (Dry matter basis)								
Wheat straw	90	3	1	38	46	12	0.3	0.1
Paddy straw	90	3	1	32	49	15	0.33	0.07
Ragi straw	90	3	1	36	52	8	-	-
Gram straw	90	6	0.5	45	35.5	13	1.0	0.08
Oil cakes (Dry matter basis)								
Mustard cake	90.0	36.0	1 1.0	10.0	33.0	10.0	0.9	1.0
Til cake	90.0	45.0	1 0.0	5.0	29.0	11.0	-	-
Groundnut cake	90.0	52.0	8.0	7.0	27.5	5.5	-	-
Cotton seed cake	90.0	23.0	9.0	24.0	37.0	7.0	-	-
Brans (Dry matter basis)								
Rice bran	90.0	12.0	1 5.0	13	45.0	15.0	0.08	1.5

Wheat bran	90.0	13.0	2.5	13	64.5	7.0	0.10	1.0
Grains (Dry matter basis)								
Gram	90.0	9.50	3.5	9.5	63.5	3.5	0.30	0.40
Maize	90.0	12.0	4.0	2.0	80.0	2.0	0.04	0.35
Barley	90.0	13.0	5.0	13	64.0	5.0	0.10	0.35
Hays (Dry matter basis)								
Indigenous grasses	85.0	5.0	1.0	50	47.0	12.0	0.3	0.20
Pasture grasses (dub etc.)	85.0	10.0	1.5	30	48.5	10.0	0.35	0.25
Leguminous hay	85.0	15.0	2.0	30	41.0	12.0	1.5	0.25
Non – leguminous fodder (on wet basis)								
Napier	25.0	2.0	0.5	10	12	1.35	0.06	0.05
Maize	25.0	2.0	0.6	8	13	1.40	0.07	0.05
Jowar	75.0	1.5	1.0	9	12	1.50	0.09	0.03
Oat	25.0	3.0	0.8	6	14	1.00	0.10	0.08
Leguminous fodder (on wet basis or as such basis)								
Berseem	15	0.5	0.5	4	4.5	3	.30	0.05
Lucerne	25	1.0	1.0	7	9	3.5	.40	0.07

Comparison of plants and animal body composition: Though the plants and animal bodies are made up of same constituents but their proportion is variable. So there are a lot of differences in animal and plant composition. In animals the major structural material is protein and minerals in the ratio of 4:1 on moisture and fat free basis which remain almost constant.

Whereas plants are made up of carbohydrates like cellulose, hemicellulose, pectin and lignin. Other differences are tabulated as:

S.No.	Parameters	Animal	Plants
1.	Major constituent	Water	Water
2.	Major organic constituent	Protein	Carbohydrates
3.	Structural component	Protein and mineral	Carbohydrates (Cellulose, Hemicellulose etc.)
4.	Reserve material	Fat (Glycogen)	Carbohydrates (Starch)
5.	Carbohydrates amount	Less	More
6.	Minerals amount	Generally constant to species	Wide variation
7.	Variation in composition	Less	Wide

Factors affecting chemical composition of plants: The chemical composition of plants depends very much upon their growth. The following factors affect the plant composition:

1. **Plant factor:** There is a marked difference in the chemical composition between the different varieties of the same species of forage because of different genetic material.

2. **Agro-climatic condition:** When a forage plant is exposed to variable agro-climatic conditions it shows variable growth performance, which directly reflects the chemical composition. The factors like atmospheric temperature and humidity affect the chemical composition of plants.

3. **Cultivation practices:** The cultivated forages, under the same agro-climatic conditions perform in different ways depending on the cultivation practices. The seed rate, seed treatment, time of sowing, method of sowing, manure and fertilizer, irrigation, weeds and disease control measures not only influence the growth and yield of the forages but also chemical composition.

4. **Stage of growth:** There is a relationship between the stage of growth of the plants and its chemical composition. The content of crude protein, soluble ash, phosphorus and potash is higher just before flowering and goes down at bloom and seed formation stage whereas, crude fibre and dry matter content increase as the plant matures. Ether extract goes down with the progressive maturity of the plant.

5. **Processing and preservation practices:** The changes in chemical composition of plants are very much influenced by method of processing and preservation. Different processing methods may change particle size, particle shape, nutrient contents and also composition of plant materials.

Biochemical basis of soil, plant and animal: The plant synthesized their feed from CO_2 and H_2O in the presence of sunlight and chlorophyll in the form of carbohydrates, which is structural as well as storage component of plants. They absorb minerals (Inorganic component) as well as water from soil and precede various biochemical reactions in plant body. Many factors like application of manures and fertilizers, irrigation, stage of growth, frequency of cutting, type of variety and strain and soil composition affect the chemical composition of the plant. As the composition of soil changes, it also affects composition of plants.

Similarly, animals utilize the plants and plant by products as their food. So composition of plants and soil also reflected into animal body composition. When plants and animals died, they are mixed into soil as a decaying organic material or as inorganic material when these are burnt. Animals also nourished the soil by their faeces, urine and other excretion and wasteproducts. Similarly plants dropped their dried leaf and fruits on the soil. So plant and animals affect the chemical composition of soil and the soil also have the same function. So there is a close inter-relationship between plants, animals and soil. And they are closely interrelated with each other. This indicates the biochemical basis of soil, plant and animals.

Q.1. Fill in the blanks:

1. A major constituent of animal and plant body is — — — —.
2. Structural component of animal body is _____ and _____. Where as plants are made up of _____.
3. _____ is the main structural components of plants where as_____ is storage component of plants.
4. There is a _____ variation in plant composition, whereas _____ Variation in animal body composition.
5. Reserve material in animal body is _____.
6. Proximate's analysis of plants was given _____ and ____.
7. Animal body was analysed by slaughter experiment technique by _____ and _____.
8. On a fat and moisture free basis animal body contain _____ percent protein and _____ percent minerals.
9. On advancing age of maturity in plants — — — — — — — — content increases.
10. Most of the straw has — — — — — percent moisture content.
11. Groundnut cake has — — — — — — — % CP and — — — — — % EE.
12. Plants synthesize complex materials from simple substances in the presence of sun light by the process of — — — — — — — — — — — — — — — — —.

Q.2. Write short notes on following.

1. Factor affecting chemical composition of plants.
2. Importance of plants composition in animal nutrition.
3. Importance of animal body composition in animal nutrition.
4. Comparison of plants and animal body composition.
5. Inter-relationship between plant, animal and soil composition.

Chapter 3

Water in Animal Nutrition

Among the nutrients indispensable (essential) for life, water ranks second only to oxygen in importance. Doubtless, water is the most important dietary essential nutrient. Loss of about $1/5^{th}$ of body water is fatal.

Water, which is composed of hydrogen and oxygen in the ratio of 2:1 is not only the largest single constituent of nearly all living plants or animal tissues but it also performs exceedingly important function. It is organic macronutrient. The water content in the plant decreases with the progressive maturity. The growing plants usually have 70 to 80 percent of water and seeds that have been thoroughly cured generally have at least 8-10 percent of water. Water content in animal body may differ due to age and nutritional status of animal.

The animal body may contain 50 to 95 percent water. In case of cattle water content is approximately 95 percent for the embryo, 75 to 80 percent at birth, 68 to 72 percent at five month and 50 to 60 percent in the mature animals. Whereas blood contains 90-92 percent, muscle contains 72-78 percent bones contain about 45 percent and enamel of teeth which is hardest tissue of body contains 5 percent water.

Functions of Water:

1. Water is an essential constituent of the animal body.
2. It is an essential part of foodstuff. It makes the food soft and palatable.
3. It helps in regulating body temperature.
4. It helps in absorption and transportation of nutrients to different parts of the body.

5. It is an essential constituent of almost all the juices and secretion of the body.

6. It helps in the excretion of waste product in the form of urine, faeces and perspiration from the animal body.

7. It acts as a solvent of many constituents of body nutrients. All the biochemical and physiological reactions take place in liquid medium.

8. It provides shape to the body cells and essential for cell nutrition. The metabolic water produced inside the body help in transportation of nutrients inside the body cells.

9. During the period of hibernation, metabolic water keeps the animal alive.

10. It helps in maintaining the acid-base balance of the body.

11. It helps in hearing by the ears and visions by the eye.

12. It acts as a cushion for tissue cells and nervous system and protects the various vital organs against shocks and injuries.

Sources of Water:

1. **Drinking water:** It is consumed by the animals from the out side source.

2. **Feed:** Moisture content of all the feeds supplies the water requirement of the animal.

3. **Metabolic / Oxidation water:** It is the water, which is produced due to metabolism of nutrients. It meets 100 percent of water requirement in hibernating animals and embryo, 5-10 percent in domestic animals and 16-26 percent in desert animals. A 100 g of each fat, carbohydrate and protein metabolism produce 107, 60 and 40g metabolic water, respectively.

4. **Bound water:** The water, which is combined with the constituents of protoplasm by either physical or chemical means. It can not separated easily from protoplasm by freezing at low temperature or by evaporation at high temperature or under dry conditions. Bound water is of special interest in connection with the ability of plants and

animals to resist at low temperature and drought condition.

Daily average water requirements of domestic animals:

Cattle	30-40 kg
Milking Cattle	30-40 kg + 1.8 kg per kg milk
Buffalo	40-50 kg
Horse	30-40 kg
Sheep, Goat and Pig	4-10 kg
Poultry	200-400 g
Rabbit	300 g
Guinea pig	30 g
Rat	6-10 g

Factors affecting water requirement:

1. **Environment:** Increased environmental temperature and humidity enhanced the water requirement in comparison to cold environment because of increased evaporative losses in hot and humid environment.

2. **Dietary factor:** High fibrous diet like dry roughages increases water requirement than less fibrous diet. Salt and uric acid excretion requires more water. So intake of salt and protein whose end product is uric acid increases the water requirement. If succulent feed is given to animals than dietary water requirement is reduced. So a 3-4 kg water per kg DMI is required for most of the animals like cattle, buffalo, horse and pig etc. whereas sheep requires 2 kg/kg DMI and poultry requires 2-3 kg/kg DMI. Young animals have higher water needs per unit of body size as compare to large animals.

3. **Animal factor:** Age, stage of growth, level of production, activity, health condition and pregnancy has a direct effect on water requirement. Other factors are salinity and sulfate content of water, temperature of water, frequency and periodicity of watering, social or behavioral interactions

of animals with environment, and other quality factors such as pH and toxic substances affect water requirement and intake. Birds require less water as compared to mammals because uric acid is the end product of protein metabolism in birds as urea in mammals.

Water metabolism: It includes absorption, homeostasis and excretion.

1. **Absorption:** Absorption takes place from all the parts of G.I.T. mainly large intestine. Organs of the digestive tract absorb most of the water ingested by an animal. A number of factors like osmotic relations inside the small intestine and nature of the carbohydrate component of the feed determine the extent to which absorption actually occurs. Water is most readily absorbed when it is taken alone as beverage, or when taken with food that after digestion forms a solution with osmotic pressure lower than that of blood plasma.

2. **Homeostasis:** It is the maintenance of uniformity and stability of water. Water balance is affected by total intake of water and losses arising from urine, faeces, milk, saliva, sweating and vaporization from respiratory tissues. It is maintained by two mechanisms.

(1) Anti diuretic hormone

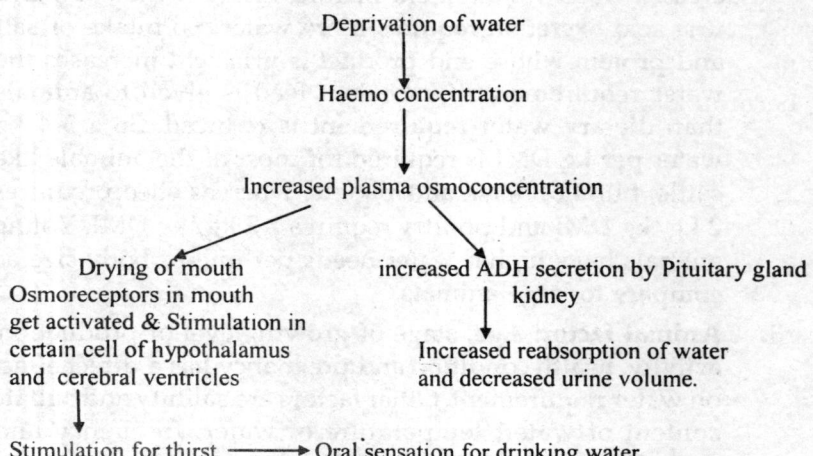

Deprivation of water

Haemo concentration

Increased plasma osmoconcentration

Drying of mouth Osmoreceptors in mouth get activated & Stimulation in certain cell of hypothalamus and cerebral ventricles

increased ADH secretion by Pituitary gland kidney

Increased reabsorption of water and decreased urine volume.

Stimulation for thirst ⟶ Oral sensation for drinking water.

(2) **Salt- appetite aldosterone mechanism:** Sodium chloride salt is an important for water retention. If NaCl decreased, water content is also decreased. Decreased Na⁺ stimulate renin synthesis which synthesize Angiotensinogen which convert angiotensin-I into angiotensin-II. Angiotensin-II promotes synthesis of aldosterone, which will act on kidney, and increased Na⁺ reabsorption, which reflects in increased water absorption and retention, and homeostasis of water, is maintained.

3. **Excretion:** Water is excreted from body by evaporation through skin, perspiration through expired air, and through faeces, urine, milk, tear and saliva. Amount lost via various routes are affected by amount of milk produced, ambient temperature, humidity, physical activity of the animal, respiration rate, water consumption and dietary factor.

Symptoms of deprivation of water: Anorexia, discomfort and inco-ordination in movement, decreased blood pressure and cardiac output, increased respiration rate, shrivelled skin, increased body temperature, delirium and death if deficiency of water continue.

Toxic elements in water: Universal solvent property of water sometime creates problems. Water can dissolve unwanted material. Such water should not be used for drinking purpose. Amount of total dissolved solids (TDS) is a measure of the usefulness of water for animals. A level of less than 3,000 mg/litre TDS can be tolerated by the animals but higher amount is harmful to animals.

Q.1. Fill in the blanks:

1. .... is the hardest tissue of body which contain — − − − − % water.

2. 100 g fats metabolism produce − − − − − −− − g metabolic water whereas 100 g carbohydrates and 100 g proteins metabolism produce − − − − − − − − and − − − − − − − −g metabolic water, respectively.

3. Loss of about — — - -- -- — — — — — part of body water is fatal.

4. Metabolic water meets out — — — — — — — % requirement in hibernating animals and — — — — — — — — — — — — % in desert animals.

5. Poultry requires — — — — — — — — — — — kg water per kg DMI.

6. Milking animals require — — — — — — — — — kg water per kg milk produced.

7. High fibrous diet — — — — — — — — — — — — — water requirement.

8. Water content in animal body may differ due to — — — — — — — — — — — — — and — — — — — — — — — — of animal.

9. — — — — % TDS (total dissolved solid) in drinking water is tolerable by animals.

10. Birds require — — — — — — — — water compared to mammals.

11. Young animals have — — — — — — — — — water needs per unit of body size than mature animals.

12. Angiotensin-II promotes synthesis of — — — — — — — — — — — — — — — .

13. Water homeostasis is controlled by two hormones viz. — — — — — — — — and — — — — — — — — — — — .

14. — — — — — — — kg water per kg DMI is required for most of the animals.

15. Bones and enamel of teeth contains — — — — — and — — — — — percent water, respectively.

Q.2. Write short notes on the following :

1. Important function of water.
2. Homeostasis of water in body.
3. Deficiency symptoms of water.
4. Factor affecting water requirements of body.
5. Differentiate between bound water and metabolic water.
6. Toxic elements in water.

Chapter 4

The Carbohydrates in Animal Nutrition

Definition of carbohydrates: Carbohydrates may be defined as polyhydroxy aldehyde, ketones or acids and their derivatives or compounds that yield these derivatives on hydrolysis. The carbohydrates are neutral chemical compounds containing the element carbon, hydrogen and oxygen, with the last two elements present in the same proportion as in water mostly, but not at all. One of the example of carbohydrate where such ratio is not found in the sugar deoxyribose ($C_5H_{10}O_4$), which is a constituent of DNA. Whereas acetic acid ($C_2H_4O_2$) and lactic acid ($C_3H_6O_3$) can be represented as hydrates of carbon but are not carbohydrates. The carbohydrates serve as both structural and reserve material in the plant. The animal body contains less than 1 percent carbohydrate, which are present in blood, muscles and liver. The carbohydrate present in animal body is also known as animal starch or glycogen.

Based upon their digestibility and solubility, the carbohydrates can be divided into two groups.

(a) Soluble carbohydrates: They are called nitrogen free extract (NFE) and include simple sugar, starch and hemicellulose, which are easily digestible in the body.

(b) Insoluble carbohydrates: They include hard fibrous substance like crude fibre, cellulose and lignin. They are less digestible by non-ruminants and easily digested in ruminants by rumen microflora and microfauna.

Functions of Carbohydrates:

1. Carbohydrates serve as a major source of energy in animal body.

2. They are essential components of production, temperature control and proper functioning of the different parts of the animal body.

3. They are essential components of milk as lactose.

4. They are stored as glycogen, excess of carbohydrates in the diet is converted into fat and stored in the fat depot. These are reserve energy materials of the body in liver and muscles of animals and starch in plants.

5. Carbohydrates are helpful in absorption of calcium and phosphorus in younger animals.

6. They help the secretion of digestive juices in gastrointestinal tract.

7. They provide suitable environment for the growth of rumen bacteria and protozoa.

8. They help in peristaltic movement of food.

9. They maintain the glucose level of plasma.

10. They are also component of several important bio-chemical compounds such as nucleic acids, coenzymes and blood group substance.

11. They play a key role in the metabolism of amino acids and fatty acids.

Classification of Carbohydrates: The carbohydrates are usually divided in to two major groups:

I. Sugars: The term sugar is generally restricted to those carbohydrates, which contain less than ten monosaccharide residues. Sugars are divided into two groups.

Sugar

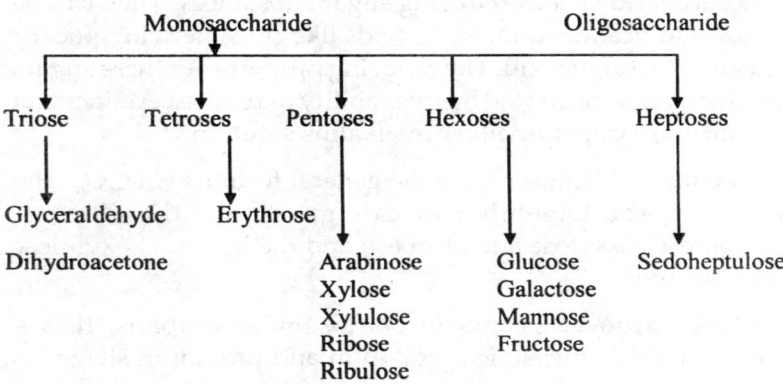

Monosaccharide   Oligosaccharide

Triose	Tetroses	Pentoses	Hexoses	Heptoses
Glyceraldehyde	Erythrose			
Dihydroacetone		Arabinose	Glucose	Sedoheptulose
		Xylose	Galactose	
		Xylulose	Mannose	
		Ribose	Fructose	
		Ribulose		

(i) **Monosaccharides:** The simplest sugars are the monosaccharides and they can not be hydrolysed into smaller units under reasonably mild conditions. They are divided into sub-groups depending upon the number of carbon atoms present in the molecules e.g. Triose ($C_3H_6O_3$), Tetroses ($C_4H_6O_4$), Pentoses ($C_5H_{10}O_5$) and Hexoses ($C_6H_{12}O_6$). The formula for the four common hexoses has been given below:

$$
\begin{array}{llll}
\text{CHO} & \text{CHO} & \text{CHO} & \text{CH}_2\text{OH} \\
\text{HCOH} & \text{HOCH} & \text{HCOH} & \text{C}=\text{O} \\
\text{HOCH} & \text{HOCH} & \text{HOCH} & \text{HOCH} \\
\text{HCOH} & \text{HCOH} & \text{HOCH} & \text{HCOH} \\
\text{HCOH} & \text{HCOH} & \text{HCOH} & \text{HCOH} \\
\text{CH2OH} & \text{CH2OH} & \text{CH2OH} & \text{CH2OH}
\end{array}
$$

(D-Glucose)   (D-Mannose)   (D-Galactose)   (D-Fructose)

Sugar containing an aldehyde (CHO) group, are classed as aldose. e.g. glucose, mannose and galactose. Whereas sugars containing a ketone group are classed as ketoses e.g., fructose.

29

Presence of active aldehyde and ketone group in monosaccharide act as reducing sugar substances. They can be oxidized to produce number of acids like gluconic acid, glucaric acid and glucoronic acid. The reducing properties of these sugars are usually demonstrated by their ability to reduce certain metal ions such as copper or silver in alkaline solution.

Pentoses: Pentoses have the general formula $C_5H_{10}O_5$. The most important member of this group are the aldoses, L-arabinose, D-xylose and D-ribose, and the ketoses, D-xylulose and D-ribulose.

L-Arabinose: Occurs in pentosans as arabans. It is a component of hemicellulose and gum and present in silage.

D-xylose: Also occurs in pentosans in the forms of xylans. These compounds form the main chain in grass hemicellulose and xylose along with arabinose produce in considerable quantities when herbage is hydrolysed with normal sulphuric acid.

D-Ribose: It is present in all living cells as a constituent of ribonucleic acid (RNA) and it is also a component of several vitamins and coenzymes.

Hexoses: Glucose and fructose are the most important naturally occurring hexose sugar, while mannose and galactose occur in plants in a polymerized form as mannans and galcutans.

D-Glucose: This sugar occurs in plants, fruits, honey, blood and other body fluid. Glucose is the major component of many oligosaccharide, polysaccharide and glucosides. In the pure state, glucose is a white crystalline and soluble in water.

Fructose or fruit sugar: It occurs free in green leaves, fruit and honey. It also occurs in disaccharides-sucrose and in fructosans. It differs from other sugars in being laevo-rotatory and also known as fruit sugar.

Mannose: It occurs in polymerized form as mannan. It does not occur free in nature.

Galactose: It is a constituent of disaccharide lactose, which occurs in milk and is also a component of gum, mucilages, pigments etc. It does not exist free in nature as Mannose.

Heptoses: Sedoheptulose is an important example of a monosaccharide containing seven carbon atoms. This heptose occurs as the phosphate, as an intermediate in the pentose phosphate metabolic pathways.

(ii) Oligosaccharides: The oligosaccharide (Oligo=few) includes all sugars other than the monosaccharides. The monosaccharides linked together with a elimination of water at each linkage and produces di, tri, tetra or polysaccharide containing 2,3,4 and large number of simple sugar molecules, respectively.

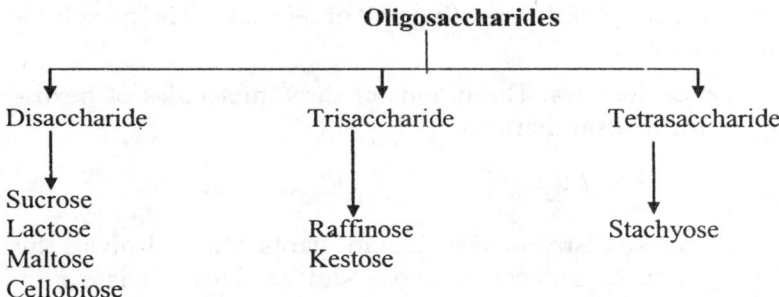

Oligosaccharides

Disaccharide	Trisaccharide	Tetrasaccharide
Sucrose		
Lactose	Raffinose	Stachyose
Maltose	Kestose	
Cellobiose		

Disaccharides: The most frequently occurring oligosaccharides in nature are disaccharides, which on hydrolysis yield two moles of simple sugar. Disaccharides consist of two molecules of hexose sugars combine together with loss of one molecules of water.

$$2C_6H_{12}O_6 \rightleftharpoons C_{12}H_{22}O_{11} + H_2O$$

The most important disaccharides are sucrose, lactose, maltose and cellobiose.

Sucrose, cane sugar, beet sugar or sacchrose: It is the familiar sugar of domestic use, widely distributed in nature and occurs in most of the plants. Sucrose is easily hydrolysed by the enzyme sucrase or by dilute acids and gives one molecule of α-D glucose and one molecule of β-D- fructose.

31

Lactose or milk sugar: It occurs in milk only as a product of mammary gland. Cow's milk contains 4.6 to 4.8 percent lactose. It is not as soluble as sucrose and is less sweet, imparting only a faint sweet taste to milk. On hydrolysis it produces one molecule of glucose and one molecule of galactose.

Maltose or malt sugar: It is produced during the hydrolysis of starch and glycogen by dilute acids or enzymes or during the germination of barley by the action of the enzyme amylase. The barley after germination and drying is known as malt and is used in the manufacture of beer and scotch malt whisky. Maltose is water-soluble but it is not as sweet as sucrose. On hydrolysis it yields two molecules of glucose.

Cellobiose: Cellobiose does not exist naturally as a free sugar, but is the basic repeating unit of cellulose. It is less soluble and less sweet.

Trisaccharides: The unions of three molecules of hexose sugars form trisaccharides.

$$3C_6H_{12}O_6 \rightleftharpoons C_{18}H_{32}O_{16} + 2H_2O$$

Raffinose distributed widely in plants. On hydrolysis this sugar produces glucose, fructose and galactose. It is a non-reducing sugar.

Tetrasaccharides: Tetrasaccharides are produce by the union of four hexose residues.

$$4C_6H_{12}O_6 \rightleftharpoons C_{24}H_{42}O_{21} + 3H_{20}$$

Stachyose is an example of tetrasaccharide, which is a non-reducing sugar, and hydrolysed to two molecules of galactose, one molecule of glucose and one molecule of fructose.

II. Non-sugars: They are tasteless, insoluble, amorphous compounds with a high molecular weight. They are divided into two sub groups.

(1) Homopolysaccharides: They are classified according to the kind of sugar, which produce on hydrolysis. For example, glucans are condensation polymer of glucose, fructans of fructose and xylans of xylose. This group of polysaccharides are a polymers of monosaccharides derivatives, such as sugar acid (eg., galacturonans) and sugar amines (e.g. glucosaminans).

(2) **Heteropolysaccharides:** They are mixed polysaccharides, which on hydrolysis yield mixtures of monosaccharides and derived products.

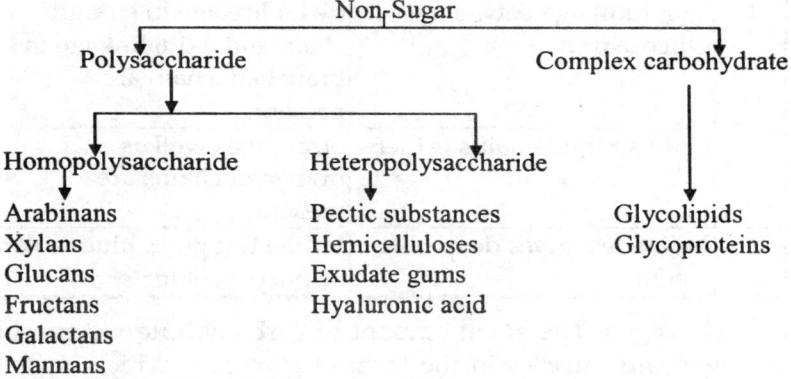

	Non-Sugar	
Polysaccharide		Complex carbohydrate
Homopolysaccharide	Heteropolysaccharide	
Arabinans	Pectic substances	Glycolipids
Xylans	Hemicelluloses	Glycoproteins
Glucans	Exudate gums	
Fructans	Hyaluronic acid	
Galactans		
Mannans		

Homopolysaccharides:

Starch: The reserve materials of most plants consist primarily of starch. When this is hydrolyzed with acids or enzymes, it is changed into dextrin, maltose and finally into glucose. In food this exists as a straight chain of glucose units called amylose, mixed with a branched chain structure called amylopectin. The quantity of amylose can be estimated in starch by a characteristic reaction with iodine, amylose produces a deep blue colour while amylopectin solution produce a blue violet or purple colour.

Amylose + Iodine ———— Deep blue colour

Amylopectin + Iodine ———— Blue violet or purple colour

Amylose is composed of linear molecules in which the - D-glucose residues are linked between carbon atom 1 of one molecule and carbon atom 4 of the adjacent molecule where as, amylopectin has a bush-like structure containing primarily -1,4 linkages but the molecule also contains side chains in which carbon atoms 6 of glucose residues is linked with carbon atom 1 of the other glucose.

Starch granules are insoluble in cold water, but when the suspension water is heated the granules swell and eventually the granule sacs rupture and a gelatinous is formed.

	Amylose	Amylopectin
1.	α- 1,4 linkage between glucose unit	α- 1,4 linkage in straight chain and α-1,6 linkage in branched chain are present.
2.	Only straight chains is there	Straight as well as branched chains are present.
3.	Iodine test gives deep blue colour	Iodine test gives blue violet or purple colour

Glycogen:. The small amount of carbohydrate reserve in the liver and muscles in the form of glycogen, which is also called "Animal starch". They form colloidal solutions, which are dextra-rotatory. Glycogen is the main carbohydrate storage product in the animal body and plays an essential role in energy metabolism.

Dextrins: These are intermediate products of the hydrolsis of starch and glycogen:

$$\left.\begin{array}{l} \text{Starch} \\ \\ \text{Glycogen} \end{array}\right\} \longrightarrow \text{Dextrin} \longrightarrow \text{maltose} \longrightarrow \text{glucose}$$

Dextrins are soluble in water and produce gum like solutions. The higher members of these transitional products produce a red colour with iodine, while the lower members do not give a colour. The presence of dextrin gives characteristics flavour to bread crust, toast and partly charred cereal foods.

Cellulose: It is glucan and is the most abundant plant constituent, farming the fundamental structures of the plant cell walls by farming chemical linkages with hemicellulose and lignin. Cellulose molecule contains between 1600 to 2700 ß-D-glucose units. Cellulose is more resistant to chemical agents than the other glucosans. On hydrolysis with strong acid glucose is produced. Enzyme produced by germinating seeds, fungi and bacteria attack cellulose and produce cellubiose, which is acted upon by enzyme cellubiase and produces glucose. It is fermented in the rumen by the microbial enzymes and produces volatile fatty acids like acetic acid, propionic acid and butyric acid.

Frutosans: It occurs as reserve material in roots, stems, leaves and seeds of a variety of plants. Fructans are hydrolysed to D-fructose and of D-Glucose. Inulin is the known polysaccharides belong to this group.

Galactans and Mannans: These are polysaccharides, which occur in cell wall of plants. It is a component of palm seeds, clovers and Lucerne.

Pectin: The term pectic substance is used to refer to a group of plant polysaccharides in which D-galacturonic acid is the main constituent in which some of the free carboxyl groups are esterified with methyl alcohol and others are combined with calcium or magnesium ions. D-galactose and L-arabinose are also present as additional components. Pectic substances are found in peel of citrus fruit, sugar beet pulp. Pectinic acid posses gelling properties and are used in Jam making.

Chitin: It is a major constituent of the exoskeleton of insects and crustacea. It is the only known example of a homopolysaccharide containing glucosamine being a linear polymer of acetyl-D-glucosamine. Next to cellulose, it is probably the most abundant polysaccharide in nature.

Heteropolysaccharide:

Hemicellulose: The hemicellulose is a group of substances, including araban, xylan and certain hexosans and polyuronides, which are much less resistant to chemical agents than cellulose. It is insoluble in boiling water but soluble in dilute alkali and hydrolyzed by dilute acids to simple sugar and uronic acid such as glucuronic and galacturonic acid.

Gum arabic: It is a useful plant gum and produced from the wound in the plant, although they may arise as natural exudates from bark and leaves. Acacia gum has long been familiar substance; in hydrolysis it yields arabinose, rhamnose and glucuronic acid.

Mucilages: Mucilages are found in few plants and seeds. Linseed mucilage produces arabinose, galactose, rhamnose and galacturonic acid on hydrolysis.

Agar: It is sulphated polysaccharides. They are found as constituents of seaweeds and in mammalian tissues. It is used as a gel-farming agent in microbial studies. Agar is a mixture of at least two polysaccharides containing sulphate ester of galactose, glucuronic acid and other compounds.

Hyaluronic acid: It is grouped under amino polysaccharides. It is present in the skin, synovial fluid and umblical cord. Solutions of this acid are viscous and play an important role in the lubrication of joints. Hyaluronic acid is composed of alternating units of D-glucuronic acid and N-acetyl-D-glucosamine. Chondroitin is chemically similar to hyaluronic acid but contain galactosamine in place of glucosamine. It is a major component of cartilage, tendons and bones.

Heparin: It is an anticoagulant, which occur in blood, liver and lung. On hydrolysis heparin yields glucuronic acid, glucosamine and sulphuric acid.

Lignin: The woody parts of plants contain a complex indigestible substance called lignin. Lignin is a high molecular weight amorphous polymer containing carbon, hydrogen and oxygen. Lignin is not a carbohydrate but because of its association with carbohydrate it is usually discussed along with carbohydrates. There is a strong chemical bonds existing between lignin and many plant polysaccharides like cellulose. Lignin is resistant to strong acids and microbial action in the rumen. It is considered to be indigestible by the animals and is responsible for poor digestion of wheat straw and paddy straw.

Carbohydrate digestion in the rumen: The major portion

of the ruminants diet consist of cellulose, hemicellulose and other carbohydrates which can not be hydrolyzed by the enzymes secreted by the animals in the digestive tract but broken down by enzymes secreted by rumen microorganisms with the production of volatile fatty acids and gases. The bacteria, which help in carbohydrate digestion, are as follows:

	Substrate		*Species*
1.	**Cellulose digester**	1.	*Bacteriodes succinogenes*
		2.	*Butyrivibrio fibrisolvens*
		3.	*Clostridium lochheadii*
		4.	*Clostridium longisporum*
		5.	*Cillobacterium cellulosolvens*
		6.	*Acetigenic rod*
		7.	*Ruminococci sp.*
2.	**Starch digester**	1.	*Clostridium lochheadii*
		2.	*Bacteriodes succinogenes*
		3.	*Butyrivibrio fibrisolvens*
		4.	*Streptococcus bovis*
		5.	*Bacteriodes amylophilus*
		6.	*Bacteriodes ruminocola*
		7.	*Succinimonas amylolytica*
		8.	*Selenomonas ruminantium*
3.	**Hemicellulose digester**	1.	*Eubacterium sp.*
		2.	*Bacteriodes ruminicola*
		3.	*Bacteriodes amylogenes*
		4.	*Ruminococcus flavefaciens*
		5.	*Ruminococcus albus*
4.	**Sugar fermenting bacteria**	1.	*Lactobacilli sp.*
5.	**Methanogenic bacteria**		*Methanobacterium ruminantium*
6.	**Proteolytic bacteria**		*All bacteria related to carbohydrate fermentation.*
7.	**Lipolytic bacteria**		*Anaerovibrio Lipolytica*

The soluble carbohydrates are rapidly fermented, starches are less rapidly fermented, whereas, the structural carbohydrates like cellulose and hemicellulose are slowly fermented. All carbohydrates are converted into pyruvic acid as shown below.

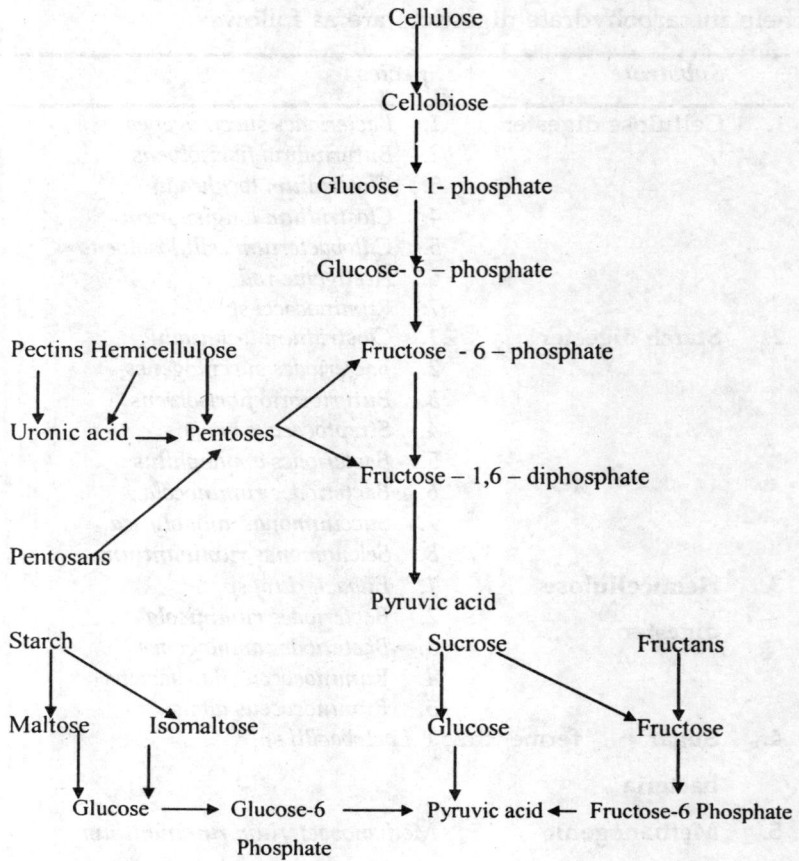

The bacteria and protozoa mainly responsible for fermentation in the digestive tract are mainly strict anaerobes although, there may be a small number of facultative anaerobes. The normal concentration of bacteria in rumen liquor is 10^{11} bacteria per ml. and protozoa are 10^6 per ml of rumen content.

Volatile fatty acid production in rumen: The feeds, which is ingested by the animals broken down to volatile fatty acids like acetic, propionic and butyric acids via pyruvic acid. Higher fatty acids like valeric and isovaleric acid etc. are also formed in smaller amounts. With normal diets the predominant acid is acetic acid followed by propionic acid and butyric acid. Volatile fatty acids represent in the following proportions.

1. Acetic acid	60-70 percent
2. Propionic acid	15-20 percent
3. Butyric acid	10-15 percent
4. Valeric and isovaleric acid	present in traces.

On an exclusive roughage diet the production of acetic acid is highest. As the concentrates in the diet are increased, the production of acetic acid reduces and that of propionic acid increases. Lactic acid is also formed as an intermediate product but is fermented to acetic and propionic acid. Mature fibrous forage give rise to VFA mixture with high proportion of Acetic acid (about 70%). Less mature forage tend to give a lower acetic acid and higher proportion of propionic acid. On concentrate feeding diet the acetic acid predominates if the rumen ciliate protozoa survive. The proportion of fatty acids production is changed under following condition:

1. High ratio of concentrates in the ration.
2. Fine ground forages,
3. Lack of physical fibrousness.
4. Green fodder low in fibre and high in soluble carbohydrates.
5. Pelleted concentrates.
6. Heated concentrates.
7. High starch diet.

This will bring relatively high ratio of propionic acid to acetic acid. The conversion of pyruate into different volatile fatty acids is shown below.

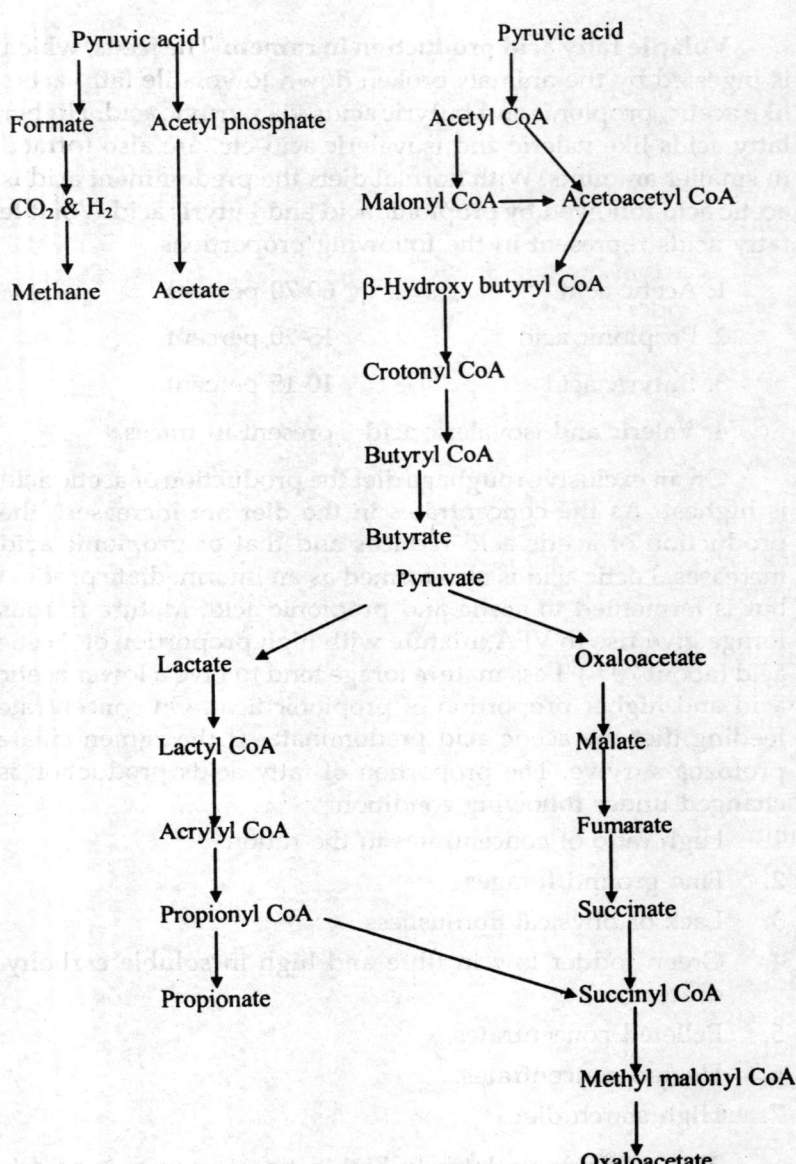

Pyruvic Acid Metabolism

Gas production in the rumen: With the fermentation of carbohydrates by the bacteria, gases are also produced. Carbon dioxide and methane at present as are principal gases. The rate of gas production in the rumen is most rapid immediately after a meal and in the cow may exceed 30 litres/hour. The typical composition of rumen gas is given below:

1. Carbon dioxide   40 percent
2. Methane   30-40 percent
3. Hydrogen   5 percent
4. Oxygen and nitrogen   (small amount ingested from air).

Carbon dioxide is produced partly as a by-product of carbohydrate fermentation and partly by the reaction of organic acid with bicarbonate of carbon dioxide by the methanogenic bacteria. Hydrogen, formate and succinate are hydrogen donors for this reaction. The quantity of methane gas formed depends upon the type of food eaten. About 4.5 g of methane is formed for every 100 g of carbohydrates fermented (digested) and the ruminant loss about 7 percent of its food energy as methane.

Most of the gases in the rumen is lost by eructation. Under metabolic disorders the gas is trapped in the rumen and the animal is unable to remove the gases and a condition known as bloat occurs.

Absorption of volatile fatty acid: Most of the volatile fatty acids are absorbed directly from the rumen, reticulum and omasum. Small amount may pass to abomasum and small intestine from where they are absorbed. Portion of these volatile fatty acids are used by bacteria and protozoa to synthesize their own polysaccharides or use as a carbon skeleton for the synthesis of their body protein.

Carbohydrates metabolism in ruminants: In ruminants considerable amounts of volatile fatty acids (Acetic, propionic and butyric acids) are produced from the carbohydrate breakdown in the rumen. The acids then pass across the rumen wall, where a little amount is converted to lactate and remaining is metabolized in the liver. The net gain of ATP per mole of acetic acid, propionic acid and butyric acids are 10, 17 and 25, respectively.

Metabolism of volatile fatty acid:

1. **Acetic acid Metabolism:** It is the major volatile fatty acid present in blood and absorbed as such. It is utilized for energy and is also a precursor of fatty acid (Short chain fatty acid of milk fat). It is never converted to glucose.

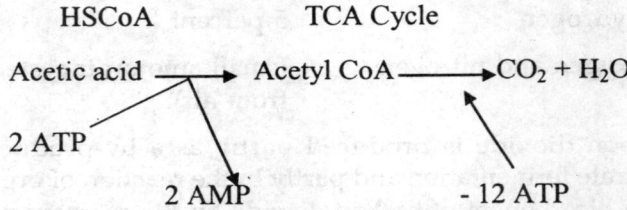

So a net 10 ATP are produced per mole of acetic acid.

2. **Propionic acid Metabolism:** Propionic acid, which is produced in rumen, is carried out to the liver where it is changed into glucose as shown below:

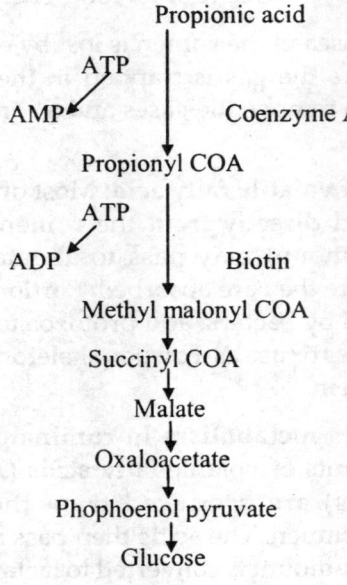

The energy balance sheet is as :-

	Mole +	ATP -
2 moles propionate to 2 moles succinyl COA	-	6
2 moles succinyl COA to 2 moles malate	6	-
2 moles malate to 2 moles phosphoenol pyruvate	6	2
2 moles phosphoenolpyruvate to 1 mole glucose	-	8
1 mole glucose to CO_2 & H_2O	38	-
	50	16

Net gain ATP per mole $\dfrac{50-16}{2} = 17$

So 17 moles of ATP are produced per mole of propionic acid.

3. Butyric acid Metabolism: It is absorbed as aceto acetic acid and b-hydroxy butyric acid in its passage across the ruminal and omasal walls. It is ketogenic in nature and utilized for synthesis of long chain fatty acid of milk fat. It is metabolised as :

Butyric acid

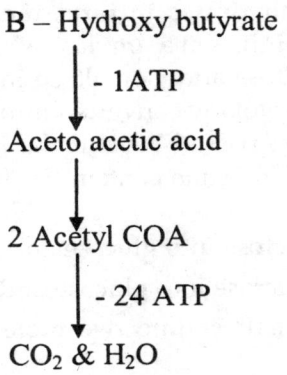

B – Hydroxy butyrate

$\Big|$ - 1ATP

Aceto acetic acid

2 Acetyl COA

$\Big|$ - 24 ATP

CO_2 & H_2O

So 25 ATP are produced per mole of butyric acid.

Digestion of carbohydrates in non-ruminants:

1. Digestion in the mouth: Here food, mixed with the saliva, which contains the enzyme ptyalin (a-amylase). This enzyme hydrolyzes starch into the maltose and isomaltose. But the food remain in the mouth for a short time and about 3 to 5 percent of the starch hydrolyzed into maltose.

The amylase enzyme hydrolzyes the a-1, 4- glucosidic bond in polysaccharide. When amylose, which contain a-1,4-glucosidic bond is attacked by a-amylase, random cleavages of these bonds give rise to a mixture of glucose and maltose. Amylopectin, on the other hand contains in addition to a-1, 4-D-glucosidic bond, a number of branched a-1, 6-D-glucosidic bonds which are not attacked by a-amylase and the product includes a mixture of branched and unbranched oligosaccharides (dextrin) in which 1, 6-D-glucosidic bonds are abundant.

2. Digestion of carbohydrates in the stomach: The action of a-amylase enzyme of saliva continues for about 30 to 50 minutes after the food has entered the stomach, that is, until the content of the fundus are mixed with the stomach secretions. Then the acid of the gastric secretion blocks the activity of the salivary amylase. The acid of the stomach juice can hydrolysed starch and disaccharides to a slight extent.

3. Digestion of carbohydrates in intestine: Pancreatic secretions contain large quantities of a-amylase which is capable of splitting starch into maltose and isomaltose in intestine. In general, the starch is almost totally converted into maltose and isomaltose before they have passed beyond the Jejunum. The epithelial cells of the small intestine contain the four enzymes *viz.*

1. Lactase, which split lactose into glucose and galactose.

2. Sucrase, which split sucrose into glucose and fructose.

3. Maltase, which split maltose into two molecules of glucose.

4. Isomaltase, which split isomaltose into two molecules of glucose.

Thus the final products of carbohydrate digestion that are absorbed into the blood are all monosaccharides. The enzyme hydrolyses starches into glucose and other carbohydrates into final products as shown below.

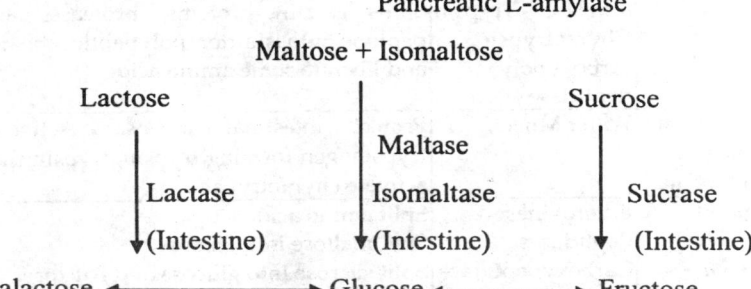

Starches

Salivary L-amylase

Pancreatic L-amylase

Maltose + Isomaltose

Lactose   Sucrose

| Maltase

Lactase   Isomaltase   Sucrase

(Intestine)   (Intestine)   (Intestine)

Galactose ←——————→ Glucose ←——————→ Fructose

Table: Digestive Juices and their function

Secretion (gland)	Principal components	Function
Saliva (Salivary gland)	Water, Mucous Salts	Soften and lubrication of food. Provide neutral medium for action of salivary amylase and help to preserve teeth against acid formed by bacteria.
	Salivary amylase	Act on starch and split into dextrin and maltose.
Gastric juice (Gastric gland)	Water, Mucous	Further soften of food. Prevent gastric juice from damaging the stomach wall.
	Hydrochloric acid	Stop the action of salivary amylase and allow pepsin to work and kills microorganisms.
	Pepsin (Secreted as a pepsinogen)	Protein moieties of the food are hydrolysed into proteases, peptone and polypeptides and curdle of milk in adults when rennin enzymes are absent.
	Rennin	Milk casein is converted into curds such as paracassinate, which is easily attached by other protein digesting enzyme.

Bile juice (Liver)	Water	Waste materials excreted with faeces or absorbed and re-excreted later.
	Bile pigment, bile salt	Alkaline therefore, neutralize acidity of chyme and stop action of pepsin but allow action of intestinal enzymes-emulsify fat.
Pancreatic juice (Pancreas)	Water, alkaline salt Prancreatic lipase Pancreatic amylase Trypsin Chymotrypsin carboxypoly peptidase	Help to increase alkalinity in intestine and combined with fatty acid to form soap splits fats into fatty acids and glycorol. Splits certain proteins, proteases and peptone into shorter polypeptide chains and liberate some amino acid.
Intestinal juice (Duodenal gland & Goblet cells)	Water Mucus	Protect intestinal mucosa. Activates trypsinogen forming trypsin, trypsin then activate chymotrypsin.
	Enterokinase Peptidases Carboxypeptidase Amino peptidase Dipeptidase, Maltase Sucrase, Lactase	Split amino acid. Split maltose into glucose. Split sucrose into glucose and fructose. Split Lactose into glucose and Galactose.

Absorption of carbohydrate in non-ruminants: The final product of carbohydrate digestion in non-ruminants is glucose, galactose and fructose. Their absorption is an active process utilizing a specific carrier protein that trans locates the molecules across the brush border membrane of small intestine. This is energy dependent process and also required Na^+ and K^+ ions. The rate of absorption of monosaccharides is also different. Galactose is fastest absorbed than glucose, fructose, mannose and slowest pentose sugar.

Factors affecting digestion of carbohydrates in non-ruminants:

1. **Particle size:** If particle size is reduced, than digestibility will be increased because of increase in surface area for digestion. Grinding broken down the cell wall so that cell contents come in contact with digestive enzymes.

2. **Form of starch:** Soluble starch is more digestible than insoluble form i.e. amylose is more digestible than amylopectin.

3. **Processing:** It improves the digestibility of starch by breaking down the cell wall. Cooked starch is more digestible than uncooked.

4. **Fibre content:** If fibre content is increased more than a level, it reduces the digestibility of carbohydrates.

5. **Enzyme Inhibitors:** Presence of enzyme inhibitors like saponin, tannins etc. reduces the digestibility of starch.

Factors affecting fibre digestibility in ruminant: Following factors affect the digestibility of crude fibre (cellulose + hemicellulose + lignin).

1. **No. and type of microbes present in rumen:** If number of microbe is more, digestibility of crude fibre increase. If cellulolytic bacteria are there, cellulose digestion is more.

2. **Relative proportion of fibre component:** If hemicellulose is more, digestibility of crude fibre is more. Lignin proportion is inversely related with fibre digestibility.

3. **Protein content in diet:** Increased protein level in diet stimulates microbial growth and improves digestibility of crude fibre.

4. **Fat content in diet:** Increased fat content in diet gives a protective layer on feed particles, which depress the fibre digestibility.

5. **NFE: CF ratio:** If NFE content is increased, then digestibility of crude fibre is decreased. Because NFE represents the soluble carbohydrates in feed i.e. starch which is a more available source of energy.

6. **Supplementation of green forages:** It stimulates digestion of crude fibre because they supply vitamins and some non-specific factors required for microbial growth.

Carbohydrates metabolism: The metabolic processes in the body are of two types. The degradation of complex compounds to simpler materials is called catabolism. Whereas those metabolic processes in which complex compounds are synthesised from simpler substances are called anabolism. As a result of the various metabolic processes; energy is made available for mechanical and chemical work. The end products of carbohydrate digestion in the simple stomach animals are glucose, galactose and fructose. Energy is produced when these are burnt to carbon dioxide and water. The energy released during metabolic processes in the cell is stored in the form of high-energy bonds particularly those found in adenosine triphosphate (ATP) and creatinephosphate (CP).

Glucose metabolism: The degradation/ synthesis of carbohydrates in the cells is done by a number of enzymes, which are mostly specific. The major pathway whereby glucose is metabolized to give energy is a two-stage process.

1. Glycolysis (Anaerobic cycle, Embden-Meyerh of Paranes pathways).

2. Tricarboxylic acid cycle (Aerobic cycle, kreb's/citric acid cycle).

1.   Glycolysis. In this process glycogen, glucose, galactose and fructose are broken down to pyruvic acid and lactic acid in the absence of molecular oxygen. The sequence of reactions is shown in the chart:

The ATP production in the glycolytic pathway: Two moles ATP are used in the initial phosphorylation of steps 1 and 3 and fructose-1-6- diphosphate so formed then break down to yield two moles of glyceraldehyde-3 phosphate. Subsequently one mole of ATP is produced directly at each step 6 and 9. Four moles of ATP produced from one mole of glucose. Since two moles of ATP are used up, the net production of ATP from ADP is two moles per mole of glucose.

Glyceraldehyde-3 phosphate is converted to 1,3 – diphosphoglyceric acid in the presence of glyceraldehyde-3-phosphate dehydrogenase enzyme and reduced NAD^+ is produced and it may be oxidised via the oxidative phosphorylation pathways, with the production of three moles of ATP per mole of reduced coenzyme. Under aerobic conditions, therefore, glycolysis yields eight moles of ATP per mole of glucose.

2. Tricarboxylic acid cycle: The next stage in the

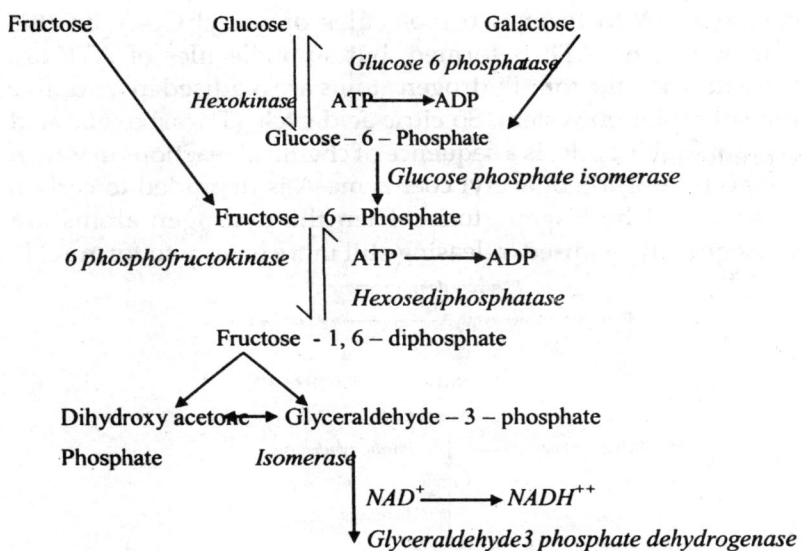

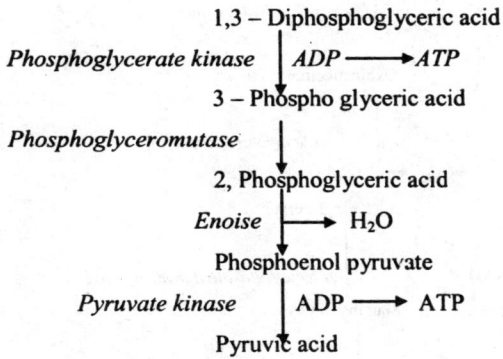

degradation of glucose is conversion of the two pyruvic acid molecules into two molecules of acetyl coenzyme A (Acetyl Co-A) as following reaction.

2 Pyruvic acid + 2 Coenzyme A= 2 Acetyl Co-A + $2CO_2$ + 4 H.

From this reaction it can be seen that two carbon-dioxide molecules and four hydrogen atoms are released, while the remainders of the pyruvic acid molecules combines with coenzyme-A to form two molecules of acetyl Co-A. In this conversion, no ATP is formed, but six molecules of ATP are formed when the four hydrogen atoms are oxidised in oxidative phosphorylation system. So citric acid cycle (Tricarboxylic acid cycle or kreb's cycle) is a sequence of chemical reactions in which the acetyl portion of acetyl coenzyme-A is degraded to carbon dioxide and hydrogen atoms. Then the hydrogen atoms are subsequently oxidised, releasing still more energy to form ATP.

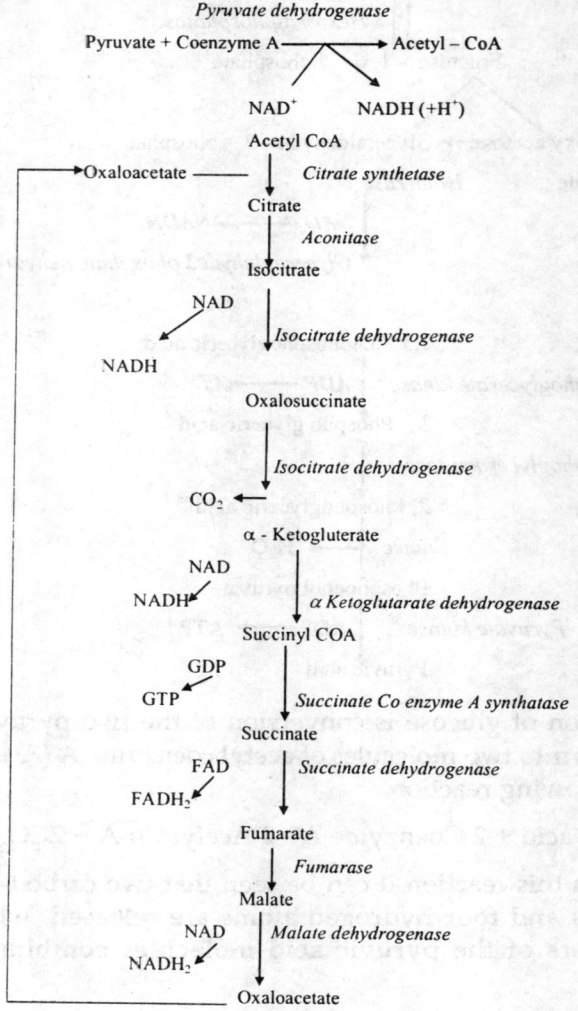

Net reaction per molecules of glucose:

$$2\,Acetyl\,Co\text{-}A + 6H_2O + 2\,ADP \rightleftharpoons 4CO_2 + 16\,H + 2\,CO\text{-}A + 2\,ATP.$$

The TCA cycle involves four dehydrogenations, three of which are NAD^+ linked and one is FAD linked, resulting in 11 moles of ATP being formed from ADP. In addition one mole of ATP arises directly with the change of succinyl coenzyme-A to succinic acid. The oxidation of each mole of pyruvate thus yields 15 moles of ATP. The total ATP production from the oxidation of one mole of glucose is given below:

1   mole of glucose to 2 moles of pyruvate produces   8
Moles ATP

2   moles of pyruvate to CO_2 and water produces   30
Moles ATP

     Total ATP per mole of glucose   =   38

Now adding all the ATP molecules formed, we find a minimum of 38 ATP molecule formed for each molecule of glucose degraded to carbon dioxide and water. Thus, 304,000 calories of energy are stored in the form of ATP, while 686,000 calories are released during the complete oxidation of each gram mole of glucose. This represents the overall efficiency of energy transfer of at least 44 percent. The remaining 56 percent of the energy become heat, which is wastage of energy.

3. Glucose metabolism by the pentose phosphate pathway: Another pathway by which glucose is metabolized within the body is the pentose phosphate pathway, the phosphogluconate oxidative pathway, and the hexose phosphate shunt. Though 95 percent or more of all the carbohydrates utilized by the muscles are degraded to pyruvic acid by glycolysis and then oxidized in the cells. The pentose phosphate pathway is of considerable importance in the liver cells, adipose tissue and the lactating mammary glands.

The steps of these pathways are shown on the following page.

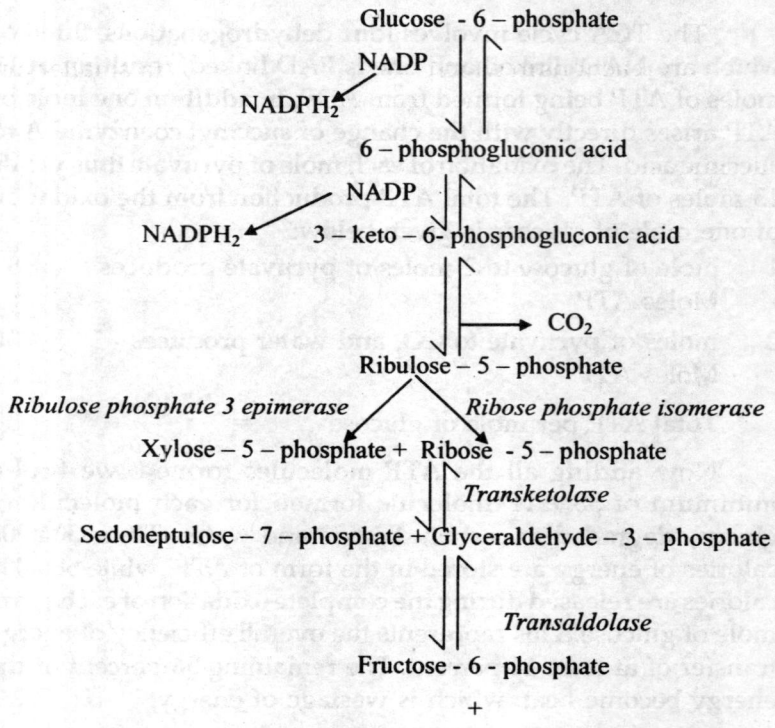

Glucose

Glucose - 6 – phosphate

NADP

NADPH$_2$

6 – phosphogluconic acid

NADP

NADPH$_2$ 3 – keto – 6- phosphogluconic acid

CO$_2$

Ribulose – 5 – phosphate

Ribulose phosphate 3 epimerase   *Ribose phosphate isomerase*

Xylose – 5 – phosphate + Ribose - 5 – phosphate

Transketolase

Sedoheptulose – 7 – phosphate + Glyceraldehyde – 3 – phosphate

Transaldolase

Fructose - 6 - phosphate

+

Erythrose – 4- phosphate

The initial phosphorylation of glucose uses 1 mole of ATP and the oxidation of hydrogen via NADP$^+$ yields 36 ATP, thereby leaving a net production of 35 ATP per mole of glucose. The efficiency of free energy captured in this case is 245000/ 686000 × 100 = 35 percent.

Net reaction

$$\text{Glucose} + 12\,NADP^+ + 6\,H_2O \rightleftharpoons 6\,CO_2 + 12\,H + 12\,NADPH$$

Gluconeogenesis: It is the process of synthesis of glucose from the sources other than carbohydrates.

When the body stores of carbohydrates decrease below normal, moderate quantities of glucose can be formed from amino acid, glycerol portion of fat, and from propionic acid. This process is known as gluconeogenesis. Approximately 60 percent of amino acids in the body protein can be converted into carbohydrates.

Glycogenesis and glycogenolysis:

Glycogen synthesis from simple sugars in the body tissues is known as glycogenesis. Glucose, galactose, fructose and mannose are readily converted to glycogen by various stages in which various enzyme systems are involved as shown below.

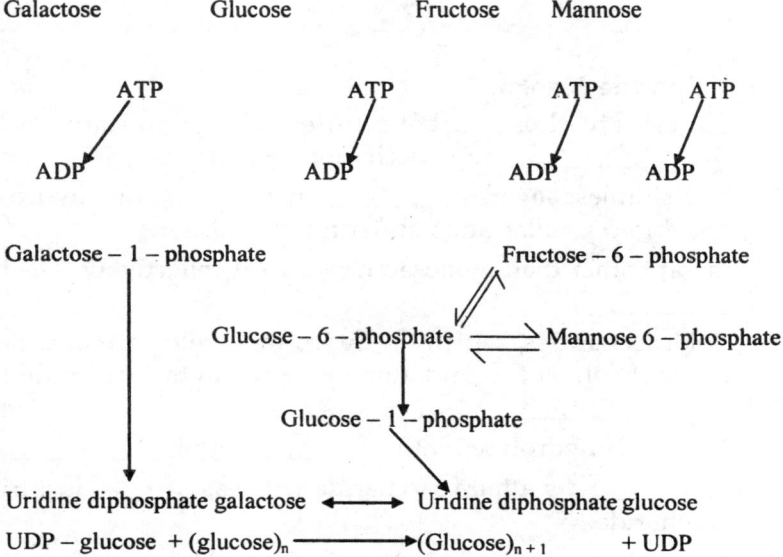

Galactose   Glucose   Fructose   Mannose

Galactose – 1 – phosphate   Fructose – 6 – phosphate

Glucose – 6 – phosphate $\rightleftharpoons$ Mannose 6 – phosphate

Glucose – 1 – phosphate

Uridine diphosphate galactose $\longleftrightarrow$ Uridine diphosphate glucose

UDP – glucose + (glucose)$_n$ $\longrightarrow$ (Glucose)$_{n+1}$ + UDP

Similarly the process of degradation of glycogen to glucose-1- phosphate in the cells is known as glycogenolysis.

Lactose synthesis: Lactose is formed by condensation of one glucose and one galactose molecule. It is formed by the action of the UDP – D – galactose with glucose in the presence of the lactose synthetase.

$$UDP - galactose + D - glucose \xrightarrow{\textit{Lactose synthetase}} UDP + Lactose$$

Fat synthesis from glucose: When the carbohydrate intake exceeds the requirement of the body for energy purposes, sugar is transformend into fat. It involves the synthesis of two components, fatty acid and glycerol, which combine with each other to give fat.

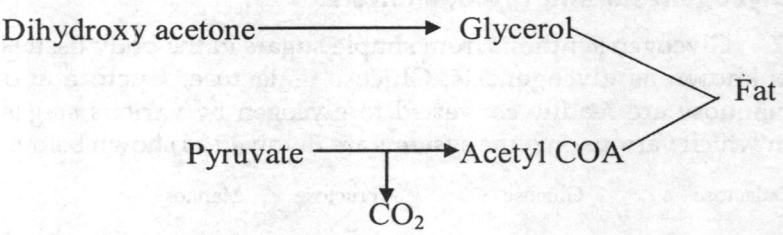

Q.1. Fill in the blanks:

1. Sugars are those carbohydrates, which contain less than_____ monosaccharide residues.

2. The simplest sugar is _____, which cannot be hydrolysed into smaller units under mild conditions.

3. Sugars other than monosaccharides are collectively called _____.

4. Polysaccharides, which on hydrolysis yield mixtures of monosaccharides and derived products, are called _____.

5. Lactose is hydrolysed into _____ and _____.

6. _____ is a tetra saccharide whereas _____ is a tri saccharide.

7. In amylose _____ linkage is found between glucose units.

8. Amylopectin has _____ linkage as well as _____ linkage between glucose unit.

9. _____ is an intermediate product of the hydrolysis of starch and glycogen.

10. Lignin contents _____ the digestibility of roughages.

11. Saliva contains an enzyme _____, which hydrolyse some part of starch into _____ and _____.

12. Lactose and sucrose sugars are hydrolysed by enzyme _____ and _____, respectively.

13. The final products of carbohydrate digestion in non-ruminants are _____, _____ and _____.

14. The absorption of galactose is _____ than glucose at intestinal level.

15. The end products of carbohydrate digestion in ruminants are _____ and _____.

16. _____ and _____ are the most commonly gases produced in rumen during carbohydrate digestion.

17. _____ is the volatile fatty acid produced in large proportion on a normal diet in ruminants.

18. Glycolysis yields _____ moles of ATP under unaerobic condition.

19. In glycolysis glucose is converted into _____.

20. The oxidation of one mole of pyruvic acid yields _____ ATP.

21. Complete oxidation of one mole of glucose yields _____ mole of ATP.

22. _____ moles of ATP are produced from one mole of acetic acid metabolism.

23. One mole of propionic acid give _____ moles ATP whereas, _____ moles are produced from butyric acid metabolism.

24. Glycogen synthesis from simple sugars in the body is known as _____.

25. Degradation of glycogen to glucose is known as _____.

26. _____ is an immediate source of energy in animal body.

27. Conversion of propionate to glucose requires vitamins _____ and _____.

28. In the horse, the large intestine in the principal site of _____ digestion

29. Lipids in the rumen are hydrolyzed & unsaturated fatty acids converted to saturated fatty acids by _____.

30. Carbohydrates, Amino acids & fatty acids are absorbed by _____ transport whereas emulsified triglycerides are absorbed by _____ diffusion.

31. Two blind-ended caeca facilitates microbial digestion in _____.

32. A process known as _____ absorbs immunoglobulins present in colostrum.

Q.2. Explain the following:

1. Classification of carbohydrates.

2. Differentiate with each other Glucose & Fructose, Lactose & Sucrose, Starch & Glycogen, Monosaccharide & Oligosaccharide, Cellulose & Hemicellulose. Homopolysaccharide & Heteropolysaccharide. Amylose and amylopectin, Glycogenesis & Glycogenolysis.

3. Explain the digestion and absorption of carbohydrates in pig.

4. Explain the digestion and absorption of carbohydrates in bullock or sheep.

5. How the carbohydrates are metabolised in non-ruminants?

6. Explain the production and absorption of volatile fatty acids in rumen.

7. How the volatile fatty acids are metabolised in goat?

8. Define the term carbohydrates. How the glucose is metabolised by glycolytic pathway?

9. Glucose is helpful for lactose synthesis and fat synthesis in the body. Justify the statement.

Chapter 5

The Protein in Animal Nutrition

Proteins are complex organic nitrogenous compounds made up of amino acids. All proteins contain carbon, hydrogen, oxygen, nitrogen and generally sulphur, many contains phosphorus. Element such as iodine, iron, copper and zinc are also occasionally present. The approximate average elementary composition of protein is as follows:

Elements	Average	percent
Carbon	50	(51-55)
Hydrogen	7	(6.5 –7.3)
Oxygen	23	(21.5-23.5)
Nitrogen	16	(15.5-18.0)
Sulphur	0-3	(0.5-2.0)
Phosphorus	0-3	(0.0-1.5)

Most proteins contain about 16 percent nitrogen, which means that the weight of protein nitrogen multiplied by 6.25 (100/16 = 6.25) equal the weight of protein. Suppose a feed sample to be analysed yields 1.0 gram of nitrogen by Kjeldahl process, then the weight of protein represented as 1.0 x 6.25 = 6.25g. Milk nitrogen is multiplied by 6.38 because milk protein contains 15.87 percent nitrogen.

Amino acids: Proteins are hydrolysed by enzymes, acids or alkalies into amino acids. About 20 amino acids are commonly found as components of proteins. Amino acids have a basic amino group and an acidic carboxyl group. So amino acids are amphoteric in nature and exist as dipolar ions or zwitter ions in aqueous solution. A pH value called isoelectric point for a given amino acid at which it is electrically neutral.

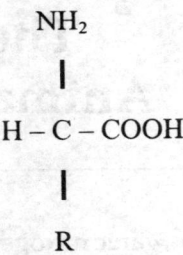

$$
\begin{array}{c}
NH_2 \\
| \\
H - C - COOH \\
| \\
R
\end{array}
$$

Classification of amino acids: Amino acids can be classified into three groups, namely, the aliphatic, aromatic and heterocyclic amino acids.

I.   Aliphatic Amino Acids

(a) Mono amino-mono carboxylic acids (Neutral amino acids)

1.   Glycine (amino acetic acid) It is simplest of the amino acids.

$$NH_2.\ CH_2.\ COOH$$

2.   Alanine (α-amino propionic acid)

$$
\begin{array}{c}
CH_3 \\
| \\
NH_2\ CHCOOH
\end{array}
$$

3.   Serine (α-amino β-hydroxy-propionic acid)

$$
\begin{array}{cc}
CH_2 \!-\! CH \!-\! COOH \\
| \quad\ | \\
OH \quad NH_2
\end{array}
$$

4.   Threonine (α-amino β-hydroxy butyric acid)

$$
\begin{array}{cc}
CH_3 \!-\! CH \!-\! CH \!-\! COOH \\
| \quad\ | \\
OH \quad NH_2
\end{array}
$$

5. Valine (α- amino-isovaleric acid)

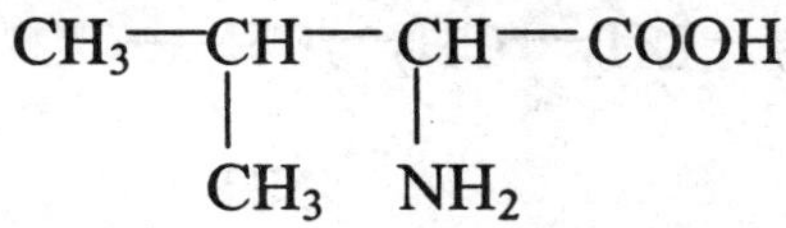

$$CH_3-CH-CH-COOH$$

with CH_3 and NH_2 substituents

$$\underset{\displaystyle CH_3 \quad NH_2}{CH_3-CH-CH-COOH}$$

6. Leucine (α-amino isocaproic acid)

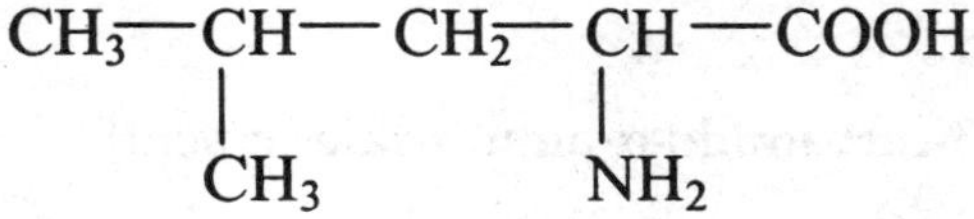

$$\underset{\displaystyle CH_3 \qquad\qquad NH_2}{CH_3-CH-CH_2-CH-COOH}$$

7. Isoleucine (α- amino β-methyl-valeric acid)

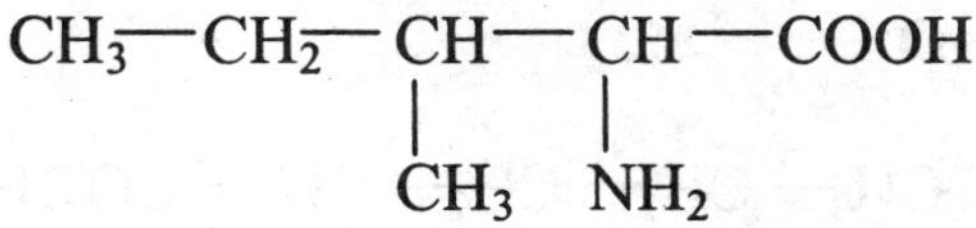

$$\underset{\displaystyle CH_3 \quad NH_2}{CH_3-CH_2-CH-CH-COOH}$$

(b) Mono-amino dicarboxylic acids (Acidic amino acids)

8. Aspartic acid (α- amino succinic acid)

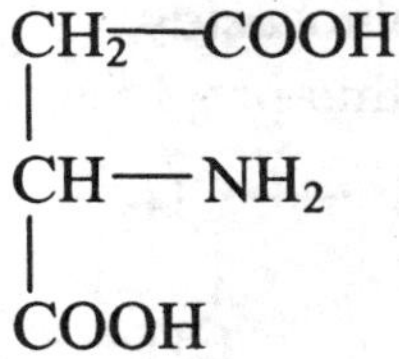

$$CH_2-COOH$$
$$|$$
$$CH-NH_2$$
$$|$$
$$COOH$$

9. Glutamic acid (α- amino glutaric acid)

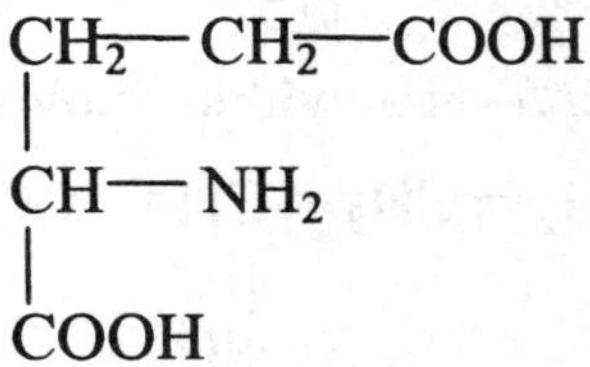

$$CH_2-CH_2-COOH$$
$$|$$
$$CH-NH_2$$
$$|$$
$$COOH$$

(c) Di-amino mono carboxylic acids (Basic amino acids)

10. Lysine (α-σ-diamino-caproic acid)

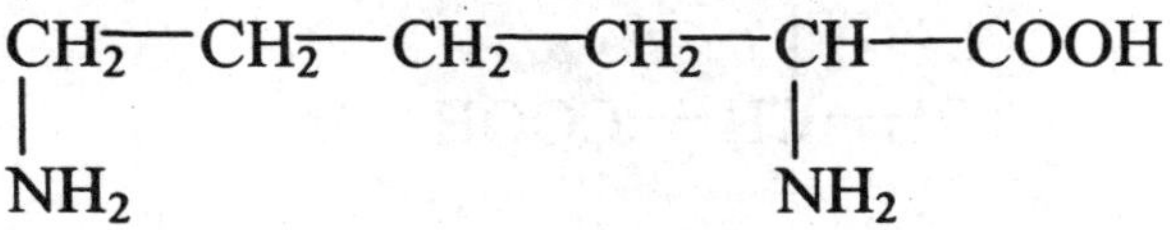

$$\underset{\displaystyle NH_2 \qquad\qquad\qquad\qquad NH_2}{CH_2-CH_2-CH_2-CH_2-CH-COOH}$$

11. Arginine (α-amino-δ-guanidine-valeric acid)

$$NH-CH_2-CH_2-CH_2-CH-COOH$$

$$C = NH \qquad NH_2$$

$$NH_2$$

12. Citrulline (δ-carbamido-α-amino-valeric acid)

$$NH_2$$

$$C = O$$

$$N - CH_2-CH_2-CH_2-CH-COOH$$

$$H \qquad NH_2$$

(d) Sulphur containing amino acids

13. Cystine (di-α-amino β-thio-propionic acid)

$$CH_2-S - S - CH_2$$

$$CH-NH_2 \qquad CH-NH_2$$

$$COOH \qquad COOH$$

14. Methionine (α-amino-γ-methylthiol butyric acid)

$$CH_3-S - CH_2-CH_2-CH-COOH$$

$$NH_2$$

15. Cysteine (α-amino-β-thio propionic acid)

$$CH_2-SH$$

$$NH_2-CH-COOH$$

II. Aromatic Amino Acids

16. Phenyl alanine (α-amino-β-phenyl propionic acid)

$$\langle\!\!\!\bigcirc\!\!\!\rangle - CH_2 - CH - COOH$$
$$\qquad\qquad\qquad |$$
$$\qquad\qquad\qquad NH_2$$

17. Tyrosine (α-amino-β-hydroxy phenyl propionic acid)

$$HO\langle\!\!\!\bigcirc\!\!\!\rangle CH_2 - CH - COOH$$
$$\qquad\qquad\qquad\qquad |$$
$$\qquad\qquad\qquad\qquad NH_2$$

III. Heterocyclic Amino Acids

18. Histidine (α-amino-β-imidazole-propionic acid)

$$CH \text{———} C \text{—} CH_2 \text{—} CH \text{—} COOH$$
$$|\qquad\qquad |\qquad\qquad\quad |$$
$$N\qquad\quad NH\qquad\quad NH_2$$
$$\quad \diagdown\!\!=\qquad\diagup$$
$$\qquad\quad CH$$

19. Proline (α-Pyrolidine-carboxylic acid)

$$CH_2 \text{————} CH_2$$
$$|\qquad\qquad\quad |$$
$$CH_2\qquad\quad CH \text{—} COOH$$
$$\quad\diagdown\qquad\diagup$$
$$\qquad\quad NH$$

20. Hydroxyproline (γ-hydroxy α-pyrolidine-carboxylic acid)

$$HO \text{—} CH \text{————} CH_2$$
$$\qquad\quad |\qquad\qquad\quad |$$
$$\qquad\quad CH_2\qquad\quad CH \text{—} COOH$$
$$\qquad\quad\diagdown\qquad\diagup$$
$$\qquad\qquad\quad NH$$

21. Tryptophane (α-amino-β-indole propionic acid)

Classification of amino acids based on charge and side chain

S.No.			
1. Non polar aliphatic amino acids			
1.	Name of A.A.	Abbreviation	Code
2.	Glycine	Gly	G
3.	Alanine	Ala	A
4.	Valine	Val	V
5.	Leucine	Leu	L
6.	Isoleucine	Ile	I
7.	Methionine	Met	M
2. Polar uncharged A.A.			
1.	Proline	Pro	P
2.	Serine	Ser	S
3.	Threonine	Thr	T
4.	Asparagine	Asn	N
5.	Glutamine	Gln	Q
6.	Cysteine	Cys	C
3. Aromatic side chain A.A			
1.	Phenyl alanine	Phe	F
2.	Tyrosin	Tyr	Y
3.	Tryptophane	Trp	W
4. Positively charged A.A.			
1.	Lysine	Lys	K
2.	Arginine	Arg	R
3.	Histidine	His	H
5. Negatively charged A.A.			
1.	Aspartic acid	Asp	D
2.	Glutamic acid	Glu	E

Function of proteins:

1. Proteins form muscles and tissues of the body; hence it is essential for the growth and development of the body.

2. They help in maintaining the loss of body tissues and muscles.

3. They help in the formation of enzymes, hormones, antigen, antibody, digestive juices of the body and regulate body osmotic pressure and acid-base balance.

4. They help in the repair of body cells as well as for the production of new cells.

5. They also supply energy to the body.

6. They are essential for the formation of egg, milk protein, wool and hairs of the animals.

7. They provide the basic cellular matrix within which the bone mineral matter is deposited.

8. Under condition of non-digestion and no-chances for denaturation, the protein accumulates inside the cells and produce toxicity. i.e. venoms of snakes and insects are infected by biting into the blood.

9. Endorphins (peptide) are found in brain and are involved in the suppression of pain.

Essential amino acid (indispensable amino acid): An essential amino acid is one needed by the animal that can not be synthesized by the animal in the amounts needed and so must be present in the protein of the feed as such.

Non-essential amino acid (dispensable amino aicd): A non-essential amino acid is one needed by the animals that can be formed from other amino acids by the animals and so does not have to be present as the particular amino acid in protein of the feed. Those amino acids which function in animal nutrition are usually classified on the basis of their essentially as follows: (in rat & man)

S. No.	Essential amino acid	Non-essential amino acids
1.	Arginine	Alanine
2.	Histidine	Aspartic acid
3.	Iso-leucine	Citrulline
4.	Leucine	Cystine
5.	Lysine	Glutamic acid
6.	*Methionine	Glycine
7.	Phenylalanine	Proline
8.	Threonine	Hydroxyproline
9.	Tryptophan	Serine
10.	Valine	Tyrosine

- **Methionine may be replaced in part by cystine.**

Chick require 10 + glycine. The pig require 9 amino acids (other than arginine)

Non protein amino acids: There are many other amino acids, which are never found as constituents of proteins but which either play metabolic roles or occur as natural products. e.g. L- Ornithine, L- Citrulline, β- alanine (in vit. Pantothenic acid), Creatine and g- aminobutyrate (in brain). L- ornithine & L- Citrulline occur in free state in the animal tissues and are metabolic intermediates in the urea cycle.

$$H_2N \; - \; CH_2 - CH_2 - CH_2 - CH - COOH$$
$$\underset{NH_2}{\big|}$$

L- Ornithine

Limiting amino acid: Livestock in definite proportions requires the essential amino acids. While the proportion may vary for different functions, it is always quite definite for any given animal performing any given set of functions. The amino acid which is present in a protein in the least amount in relation to be animal's need for that particular amino acids can be used by the animal toward meeting its essential amino acid requirement only to the extent that the so-called limiting amino acid is present. It will be noted that lysine is the limiting essential amino acid of corn.

Structure of proteins: The structure of proteins can be considered under four basic headings:

1. **Primary Structure:** Proteins are built up from amino acids means of a linkage between the α-carboxyl of one amino acid and the α -amino group of another acid. This type of linkage is known as the peptide linkage. Large number of amino acids can be jointed together by this means with the elimination of one molecule of water at each linkage to produce poly peptides. The term primary structure refers to the sequence of amino acid along the polypeptide chains of protein.

2. **Secondary Structure:** In secondary structure the peptide chain exist in the form of a right-handed -helix. The spiral is stabilized by hydrogen bonding between the amino (NH) and carbonyl (CO) group of adjacent amino acids.

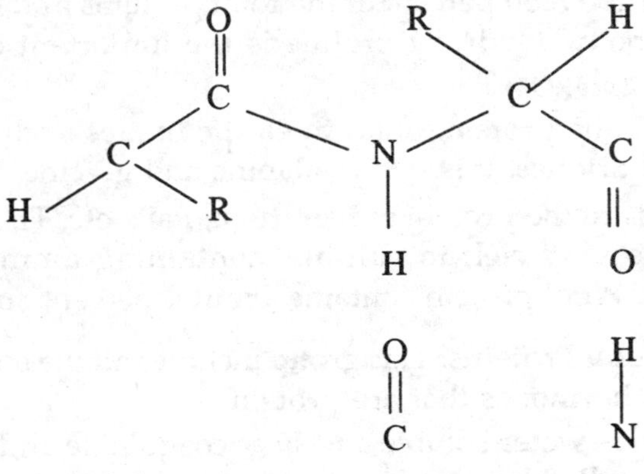

3. **Tertiary structure:** It describes how the chains of the secondary structure further interact through the R-groups of amino acid residues. These interaction causes folding and bending of the polypeptide chain, the specific manner of the folding giving each protein its characteristics biological activity. The tertiary structure is stabilized by H-bonding, S-bonding (disulphide linkage), self bridge between basic amino acid and acidic amino acids and certain amino acids like alanine, phenylalanine and valine in which R-group is non-polar. If it is coiled all non- polar amino acids come in contact to form a hydrophobic centre.

4.   Quaternary Structure: Protein poses quaternary structure if they contain more than one polypeptide chain. The force that stabilized these is hydrogen bonds and electrostatics or salt bonds formed between residues on the surface of the polypeptide chain.

Classification of proteins: Proteins may be classified into three main groups according to their shape, solubility and chemical composition.

I. Fibrous Proteins: These proteins are insoluble and very resistant to animal digestive enzymes. They are composed of elongated, filamentous chains, which are joined together by cross linkages. They are as follows:

1.   Collagens are the main proteins of connective tissues. It makeup about 30 percent of the total proteins in the mammalian body. Hydroxy proline is the important component of collagens.

2.   Elastin is the protein found in elastic tissues such as tendon and arteries. It is rich in alanine and glycine

3.   Keratins are the protein of hair, hoof, nails etc. These proteins are very rich in sulphur containing amino acid, cystiene. Wool protein contains about 4 percent sulphur.

II. Globular Proteins: This group includes all the enzymes, antigens and hormones that are protein.

1.   Albumin is water-soluble and heat coagulable and occurs in eggs, milk, blood and many plants.

2.   Globulins are present in eggs, milk and blood and are the main reserve protein source in seed.

3.   Histones are basic protein, which occur in cell nucleus where they are associated with DNA. They are water-soluble but not heat coagulable, and on hydrolysis yield large quantities of histidine and lysine.

4.   Protamines are basic protein of relatively low molecular

weight, which are associated with nucleic acid and are found in large quantities in the nature, germ cells of vertebrates. Protamines are rich in arginine.

III. Conjugated Proteins: Conjugated proteins are composed of simple protein combined with some non-protein substances as prosthetic group.

1. Phosphoprotein is the protein which on hydrolysis yields phosphoric acid and amino acids. Casein of milk and phosvitin of egg yolk are the best known phosphoproteins.

2. Glycoproteins are conjugated proteins with one or more heterosaccharides as prosthetic groups. In most of the glycoproteins, glucosamine or galactosamine or both, in addition galactose and mannose may be present. Glycoproteins are components of mucous secretions which act as lubricants in many parts of the body eg. ovalbumin.

3. Lipoproteins are proteins conjugated with lipid lecithin and cholesterol. They are the main components of cell membranes and play a basic role in lipid transport.

4. Chromoproteins contain pigment as a prosthetic group. Examples are haemoglobin, haemocyanin, cytochrome and flavoproteins.

5. Nucleoproteins are compound of high molecular weight and conjugated with nucleic acid.

6. Metalloproteins a large group of enzyme proteins contain metallic elements, such as Fe, Co, Mn, Zn, Cu, Mg, etc. which are essential part of these proteins.

IV. Derived Proteins: This class of proteins includes those substances formed from simple and conjugated proteins.

1. **Primary derived proteins:** If there is a slight change in the proteins molecules such as metaproteins and coagulated proteins, they are called primary derived proteins.

2. **Secondary derived proteins:** If there is a large change in protein structure, they are called secondary derived proteins. They are precipitated by phosphotungstic acid. The examples are proteoses, peptones and peptides.

Non-protein Nitrogenous compounds: Nitrogenous compounds, which are not classed as proteins occur in plants and animals called as non-protein nitrogenous compounds. Amino acids like glutamic acid, aspartic acid, alanine, serine, glycine and proline forms the main parts of the non-protein nitrogenous fraction in plants, Other compounds are nitrogenous lipids, amines, amides, purines, pyrimidines, nitrates and alkaloids. In addition many members of the vitamin B-complex contain nitrogen in their structure.

Nucleic acid: Nucleic acids are high molecular weight compounds which, on hydrolysis, yield a mixture of basic nitrogenous compound (purines and pyrimidines) a pentose (ribose and deoxyribose) and phosphoric acid. They play a fundamental role in living organism as a store of genetic information and synthesis of proteins. Nucleotide containing ribose is termed as ribonucleic acid (RNA) while those containing deoxyribose are referred as deoxyribonucleic acids (DNA).

Nucleosides and Nucleotides: They are carbohydrates derivatives in which purines and pyrimidines found in nucleic acids are linked to a sugar in a ß-N-glycosyl bond. The sugar is either D-ribose or deoxyribose in the naturally occurring nucleoside. If the nucleosides such as adenosine are esterified with phosphoric acid, they form nucleotides. Naturally occurring nucleotides are adinosine monophosphate (AMP), adinosine diphosphate (ADP) and adinosine triphosphate (ATP).

Digestion of protein in non-ruminants: There is no digestion of protein in the mouth because saliva has no proteolytic enzyme. But saliva softens the food particles, which is helpful for ingestion of protein.

Digestion of proteins in the stomach: The digestion of protein start in the stomach by the action of peptic enzymes. Pepsin and gastricin are the most important peptic enzymes of the stomach. Both enzymes are most active at about pH 2 to 3, and completely inactive at pH above 5. Gastric glands secrete hydrochloric acid at a pH of about 0.8, but by the time it's mixed with the stomach contents, the pH ranges around 2-3, a high favourable for peptic enzyme activity. These enzymes are capable of digesting protein, collagen and nucleo proteins into proteoses, peptones and polypeptides.

Digestion of proteins in the intestine:

1. Digestion of proteins by pancreatic secretions: When the proteins leave the stomach they ordinarily are in the forms of proteoses, peptones, large polypeptides and amino acids. Immediately upon entering the duodenum the partial breakdown products are attacked by the pancreatic enzymes trypsin, chymotrypsin and carboxpolypeptidases. These enzymes are capable of hydrolyzing all the partial breakdown products of proteins to polypeptides and amino acids.

· 2. Digestion of polypeptides by the epithelial enzymes of the small intestine:

The epithelial cells of the intestine contain several different enzymes for hydrolyzing the final peptide linkages of the different dipeptides into amino acids. So the end product of protein digestion is various amino acids.

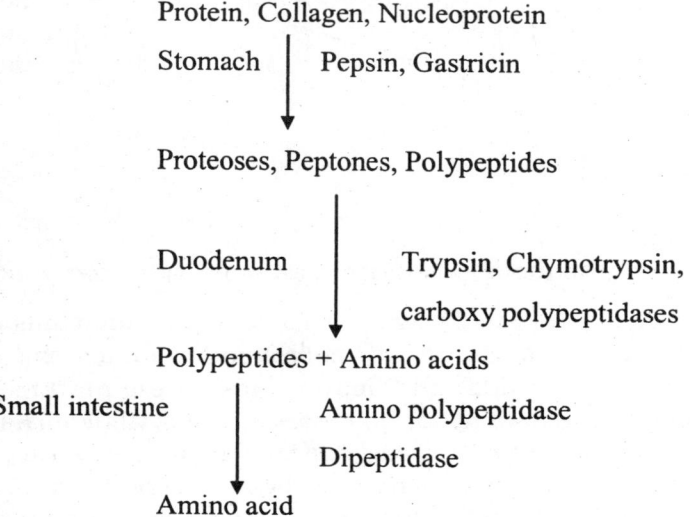

69

Digestion of protein in Ruminants: The digestion and metabolism of proteins in ruminants are different than non-ruminants. The biological success of the ruminant in utilizing crude proteins and non-protein nitrogenous (NPN) substances seems to be dependent upon the physiological regulation of rumen environment as microbial habitat. As the microbes multiply, they synthesize protein to construct their own bodies by utilizing dietary protein and NPN substances. This microbial protein is available to the host for subsequent digestion in the lower part of the gut.

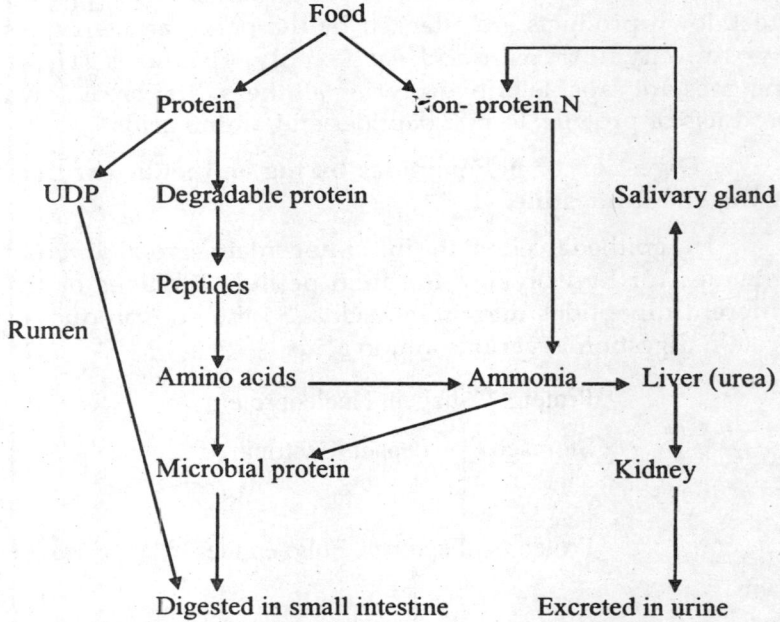

Digestion and metabolism of protein and NPN compound:

Proteolysis: The proteins available to the ruminants are digested by the process of proteolysis in the rumen and are converted to peptides and amino acids. These are further fermented, by deamination to carbon dioxide, ammonia and short chain fatty acids. Ruminal proteases are mainly cell bound but may be located on the surface of the cell where the substrate is freely accessible to the enzymes. These proteolytic enzymes are rather non-specific in their character, since their ability to ferment a range of proteins is not influenced by changes in the microflora brought about by different rations. It appears that for the bacterial proteases to act efficiently the protein must be in solution farm. Different proteins are proteolysed at different rates and rate of digestion of a particular protein is fairly constant. The rate of proteolysis is closely related to solubility of proteins in the water and in salt solution resembling rumen fluid.

In spite of a strong proteolytic activity in the rumen, the amino acid concentration in rumen fluid is low because of the presence of microbial deaminases, the activity of which increases with increasing protein content of the ration. The enzyme is directly responsible for the process of deamination.

Ammonia production: The ammonia in rumen liquor is the key intermediate in the microbial degradation and synthesis of protein. Parts of the ammonia produced in the rumen liquor is utilized by the rumen bacteria along with carbon moiety to synthesize the microbial proteins, and excess of ammonia is absorbed into the blood, carried to the liver and converted to urea. Some of this urea may be returned to the rumen via the saliva, and also directly through the rumen wall, but the larger part is excreted in the urine and thus wasted out. The rumen fluid has a pronounced urease activity so that urea entering it is rapidly hydrolysed to ammonia and carbon dioxide. Increased quantity of readily fermentable sugars decrease the concentration of ammonia in the rumen thereby helping better utilization of proteins and non-protein nitrogen.

Fate of ammonia: Rumen microbes for their rapid multiplication utilize considerable protein and utilize ammonia and fix it as excellent body protein composing of essential and non-essential amino acids in presence of soluble carbohydrates, particularly starch. The rumen microbes continuously passes to the abomasum and small intestine, their cell proteins are then digested by usual gastric enzymes of the abomasum and are absorbed as units of amino acids mostly in the region of the small intestine. A portion of the total ammonia of the rumen is absorbed in to the systemic blood and converted into urea in the liver.

Urea recycling: It is now well established that blood urea enter back into the rumen directly by transfusion through rumen wall and also indirectly through saliva. The process would be of great value to animals on low nitrogen intake.

Microbial protein synthesis: Microbes in the rumen degrade large proportion of dietary proteins and utilize some of the degradation products for their own protein synthesis. These microbes can also make use of NPN compound and can upgrade the dietary protein of low biological values into microbial proteins of high biological values. Therefore, it would be advantageous to feed poor quality protein and NPN compound to the ruminants.

Utilization of non-protein nitrogen compound: Ruminants can utilize non-protein nitrogenous compound as a source of protein through the microorganisms. The compound which are commercially available are urea and biuret etc. as a source of NPN compounds for ruminants. First evidence of NPN compounds used in animal feed in Germany in 1879. Finger ling *et al.* 1937 produced clear evidence that urea can utilized to supply a part of protein needs for growth of ruminants. Urea is very common and now it has been accepted that urea can replace about 30 to 40 percent of DCP requirement.

$$NH_2CONH_2 \xrightarrow[\text{Hydrolysis}]{+H_2O \ \text{Urease}} 2\,NH_3 + CO_2$$

Urea

Urea is white crystalline, deliquescent solid. Pure urea has nitrogen content 464-466 gram/ Kg (2900-2913 gram CP/Kg) Urea entering the rumen is rapidly hydrolyzed to ammonia and carbondioxide by bacterial urease enzyme. This ammonia is used as a nitrogen source by the rumen microorganisms for synthesis of microbial protein along with the carbon skeleton coming from the carbohydrates/proteins. Efficient utilization of ammonia for microbial protein synthesis requires the optimum initial ammonia concentration and a readily available source of energy for protein synthesis. Feeding practices intended to meet these conditions include mixing urea with other feeds which should be low in rumen degradable protein and high in readily fermentable carbohydrates. It is important to avoid accidental over consumption of urea since the subsequent rapid absorption of ammonia from the rumen can exceed the ability of the liver to re-convert it to urea, hence causing the ammonia concentration of peripheral blood to reach toxic level. Optimum level of ammonia in rumen is 5-8 mg/100 ml. Ammonia concentration is increased beyond the optimum level when diet protein is more than 13%. Urea become toxic if the level of ammonia exceeds 80 mg/ 100 ml of rumen liquor and 1 mg per 100 ml of blood. Whereas, 3 mg per 100 ml of blood ammonia concentration is fatal. To avoid ammonia toxicity, not more than $1/3^{rd}$ of the dietary nitrogen should be provided as urea. Urea does not provide the source of energy, minerals and vitamins. Urea is also deficient in sulfur containing amino acids so as a source of sulfur, 0.13 gram anhydrous sodium sulfate is added per gram of urea.

Derivatives of urea have been used for animal feeding with the intention of retarding the release of ammonia. Biuret is produced by heating urea. It is colourless crystalline compound. Biuret has nitrogen content 408 gram/Kg (2550 gram CP/Kg). Nitrogen in biuret is not readily utilized as protein source. Biuret is non toxic even at higher levels. Biuret is less rapidly hydrolysed than urea but requires a period of several weeks for rumen microbes to adapt to it. Adaptation becomes fast if rumen liquor innoculation with rumen liquor from an adopted rumen. However, neither biuret nor isobutylidene diurea nor urea- starch compounds have consistently proved superior to urea itself. Uric acid, which is present in poultry faeces, is also used as ruminant feed.

Urea toxicity symptoms: Nervousness, muscle tremors, difficulty in respiration, excessive salivation, bloat, tetany, convulisons and death within 2 to 3 hours are the symptoms of urea toxicity. The severity of symptoms depends upon the dose of urea intake. The drenching of glacial acetic acid cold water is the line of treatment in urea toxicity. To avoid urea toxicity, urea should be mixed properly in the feed and level of urea should be 3 percent in the concentrate mixture or 1percent in the sole ration of ruminants. Whereas BIS recommended 1 percent of urea in the concentrate mixture of ruminants.

Utilization of NPN substance by non-ruminants: Non-ruminants are also able to utilize NPN compound for the synthesis of non-essential amino acids and the optimum level is 0.3 percent of the diet. But NPN substances are of little practical value for non-ruminants. It is ineffective for swine but used to some extent by mature horses on low protein diet and by hen fed diets well balanced in the essential amino acid.

Protein metabolism: Dietary proteins are digested through the action of proteolytic enzymes to amino acids. These amino acids are absorbed through the small intestine into the portal blood. Major site of absorption of amino acids is proximal $2/3^{rd}$ of small intestine. Absorption is an active type in which transport of sodium is involved. Tripeptides are absorbed more rapidly than dipeptides, which are in turn faster than free amino acids. There is a competition for absorption within groups of free amino acids, viz, acidic, basic, neutral and imino acids but no competition between groups which suggests that slightly different mechanisms of transport exist for different chemical configurations. They are transported to the liver and then to the systemic blood circulation. Amino acid of the blood pool serves as a major source for tissue protein synthesis. Excess of amino acids, which are not required for synthesis of tissue protein, hormones, enzymes etc. are catabolized in the liver tissues. The catabolism of amino acid involves deamination whereby ammonia and a-keto-acid are formed. The released ammonia is converted into urea or may be utilized by a-keto acid to form amino acid.

Amino acid degradation take place mainly in the liver although, the kidney shows considerable activity, unlike muscular tissues which is relatively inactive.

1.   Deamination: Separation of nitrogen from an amino acid in the form of ammonia and the detachment of non-nitrogenous residue from it, is called deamination. The nitrogen become useless during this process but the non-nitrogenous portion serves as a source of energy to the animal body. With the result of oxidative deamination of all the amino acids there is formation of ammonia and the non-nitrogenous residue keto-acid.

$$+ H_2O + NAD^+$$

Alanine $\longrightarrow$ Pyruvic acid + Ammonia + NADH

Alanine dehydrogenase

$$+ H_2O + NAD^+$$

Glutamic acid $\longrightarrow \alpha$-ketoglutamic acid + Ammonia + NADH

Glutamic dehydrogenase

The ammonia thus, liberated is converted to urea by the liver and excreted through urine from the body. The non-nitrogenous portion serve, as a energy source which either follow the pathways carbohydrate metabolism or fat metabolism.

Non oxidative deamination: These reactions are catalyzed by amino acid dehydratase and also require vitamin B_6.

Serine $\longrightarrow$ Pyruvate + NH_4^+

Threonine $\longrightarrow \alpha$ - Ketoglutarate + NH_4^+

Asparatic acid $\longrightarrow$ Fumaric acid + NH_4^+

3.   Transamination: In transamination the amino group of one amino acid is transferred to the a-carbon atom of a keto acid, resulting a production of another keto acid and amino acid. The reactions are catalysed by enzyme known as amino transferases. The reaction for aspartic acid may be represented as follows:

Aspartic acid

Aspartic acid + α-ketoglutaric ⇌ Oxaloacetic acid + Glutamic acid.

acid   Transferases

Transaminase

Pyruvic acid + Glutamic acid ⇌ Alanine + α-ketoglutaric acid

In this way the pyruvic acid which is a product in the carbohydrate metabolism is transferred to amino acid by the process of transamination and serves in protein synthesis in animal body.

Transmethylation: This is the process by which methyl group is transferred from the amino acid methionine and joins the some other compounds to form choline for the formation of creatinine or phospholipid.

Urea formation: One of the consequences of amino acids metabolism is the production of ammonia, which is highly toxic. Some of this may be used in the amination of amino acids synthesis in the body. Most is excreted from the body, as urea in mammals and uric acid in birds.

The formation of urea which take place in the liver involve two stages both of which require an energy supply in the form of ATP. The first step is the formation of carbamoyl phosphate from CO_2 and NH_3 in the presence of carbamoyl phosphate synthetase

$$CO_2 + NH_3 + H_2O \longrightarrow Carbamoyl\ phosphate$$
$$2\ ATP \qquad 2\ ADP$$

The carbamoyl phosphate then react with ornithine to yield citrulline, which finally converted into urea and ornithine via kreb's urea cycle.

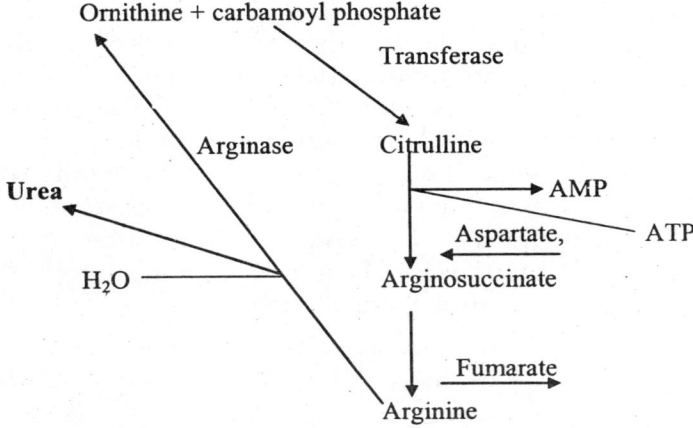

Ornithine + carbamoyl phosphate
Transferase
Arginase
Citrulline
Urea
AMP
Aspartate,
ATP
H_2O
Arginosuccinate
Fumarate
Arginine

Utilisation of amino acids: The absorbed amino acids in the body are utilised for various functions.

1. For the protein synthesis
2. For the synthesis of essential amino acids
3. As a source of energy and ammonia
4. For a special function - various important compounds are formed from amino acids which are very helpful in living system.

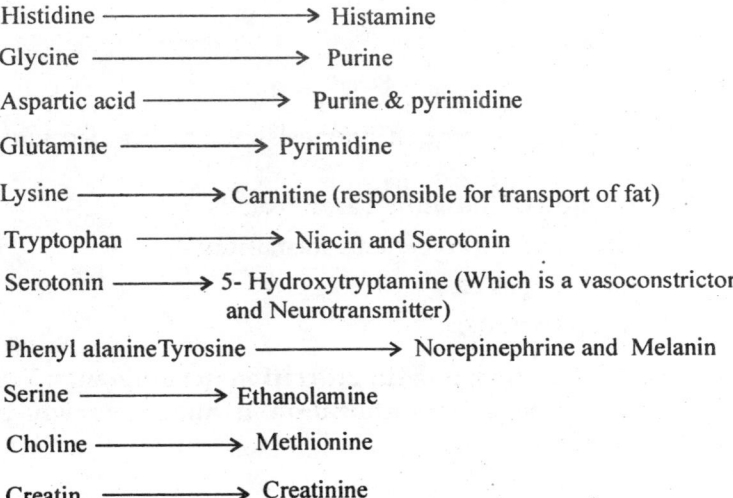

Histidine ⟶ Histamine

Glycine ⟶ Purine

Aspartic acid ⟶ Purine & pyrimidine

Glutamine ⟶ Pyrimidine

Lysine ⟶ Carnitine (responsible for transport of fat)

Tryptophan ⟶ Niacin and Serotonin

Serotonin ⟶ 5- Hydroxytryptamine (Which is a vasoconstrictor and Neurotransmitter)

Phenyl alanineTyrosine ⟶ Norepinephrine and Melanin

Serine ⟶ Ethanolamine

Choline ⟶ Methionine

Creatin ⟶ Creatinine

Protein synthesis: Proteins are synthesized from amino acids, which become available as the end products of digestion or as the result of synthetic processes within the body. Direct amination may take place as in the case of a- ketoglutarate, which yields glutamate. The glutamate may undergo further amination to give gluatmine and undergo transamination reactions with various keto acids to give amino acids. Amino acids other than glutamate may undergo such transaminations to produce new amino acids. Thus both alanine and glycine react with phosphohydroxypyruvate to give serine.

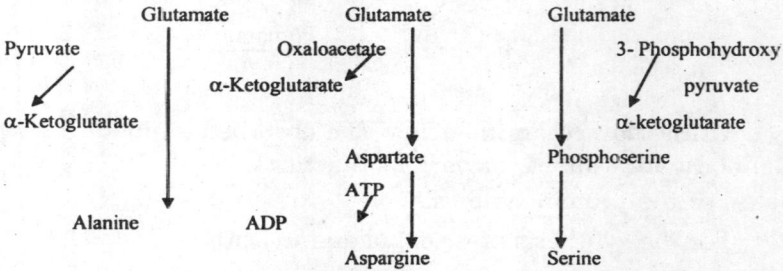

Amino acid Synthesis from glutamate.

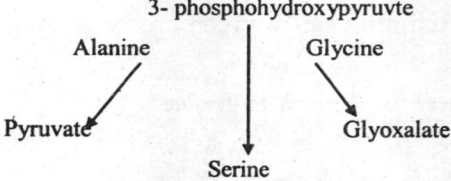

The process of protein synthesis may be divided into four stages:

1. Activation of individual amino acids
2. Initiation of peptide chain formation
3. Chain elongation
4. Chain termination.

Factor affecting protein utilization in ruminants: Various factors affect the protein utilization in ruminants, which are described below.

1. **Dietary level of protein:** Protein utilization is improved by increasing the level of protein in the diet upto the level of requirements however, more protein supplement above the requirement is not properly utilized.

2. **True protein nitrogen (TPN) vs. Non-protein nitrogen (NPN) ratio:** True protein is the best source of nitrogen which is followed by mixture of TPN + NPN and than NPN. However, NPN utilization will depends on the degradability of dietary protein, availability of keto acid for amino acid synthesis and minerals specially sulphur.

3. **Degradability of protein:** Protein utilization is decreased as the degradability of protein in rumen is increased. The optimum ratio of rumen degradable protein (RDP) and rumen undegradable protein (RUP) in high yielding animals is 40: 60. Degradability of different feed is different.

Feed	Degradability (percent)
Urea	100
Casein	90
Barley	80
Groundnut	60
Maize	40
Fish meal	30

Fish meal is least degradable in rumen. So fish meal gives better quality protein for ruminants. Fish meal is called naturally protected protein because it is 70 percent undegradable, which reach to lower GIT as such and provide high quality protein.

4. Indigestible nitrogen content in diet: Indigestible nitrogen present in feed is due to damage of protein. Excessive heating leads to browning of protein in which epsilon amino group of amino acid lysine combine with cellulose and hemicellulose to form complex which is insoluble in acid detergent solution. So it is called acid detergent insoluble nitrogen (ADIN) or artifact lignin. High level of indigestible nitrogen in diet reduces the protein utilization.

Protein deficiency Symptoms: It includes reduced feed intake and utilization, reduced growth rate, infertility, reduced serum protein concentration, accumulation of fat in the liver and carcass, reduced synthesis of certain enzymes and hormones resulting depression of most metabolic activities which may lead even to early death.

The classical disease of protein malnutrition of the young is kwashiorkar. The marasmus is a calorie deficient state. The general term for both the conditions in protein/calorie malnutrition (PCM) which is characterised by low blood protein level, poor digestion, lethargic patient and depressed immune system.

Amino acid deficiency: It is a condition in which the dietary supply of one or more of the essential amino acids is less than that required for the efficient utilization of other amino acids and other nutrients. Diets are in general unlikely to be completely devoid of any one or more amino acids but may be deficient in respect of required quantity. The amino acid, which provides the lowest proportion of the theoretical requirement, is referred to as the first limiting amino acids (Lysine).

Amino acid imbalance: This term is normally restricted to circumstances where the composition of essential amino acids in the diet results in a further poorer animal performance than would be expected in case of amino acid deficiency where the effect depends on the extent of limiting amino acids. Imbalance is produced by the addition to a diet low in total protein of either the second limiting amino acid, or more usually a group of amino acid which doesn't include the first limiting amino acid. The adverse effect on performance can be avoided by supplementation with the first limiting AA.

Amino acid antagonism: Certain amino acid interferes the metabolism of other amino acids eg. Lysine in excess increases the excretion of Arginine. Excess lysine also increases the activity of arginase enzyme and arginine is broken down to urea and ornithine. Antagonism differs from imbalance in that the supplemented amino acids need not be limiting amino acid.

Secondly it refers to an excessive amount of amino acid in the diet which affects only those amino acids belonging to members of the structurally similar group.

Amino acid toxicity: The term amino acid toxicity is used when the adverse effect of an amino acid in excess cannot be over come by supplementation with other amino acids. The effect of the inclusion of the gross amounts of an individual amino acid with in a diet varies among amino acids. Threonine, even in a very large amount (50g/kg of the DM of the diet) is tolerating well and causes only a moderate depression of feed intake and growth. Tyrosine, however when ingested in large amounts by young growing rats gives a low protein diet, not only depress severely feed intake and growth but caused severe eye and paw lesions, and in great excess is lethal. Methionine is the most toxic and in amounts exceeding 20 g / kg of the dry matter of the diet may produce severe histopathological changes.

Q.1. Fill in the blanks:

1. All proteins contain on an average about — — — — — — — — % nitrogen.

2. An amino acid, which is not synthesised by the animals in the required amount, is called — — — — — — — — —.

3. Linkage between different amino acids is called — — — — — — — —.

4. Sulphur containing amino acids are — — — —, — — — — — — and — — — — — —.

5. Aromatic amino acids are — — — — — — and — — — — — — —.

6. Neutral amino acids are — — — — — — —, — — — — — — — —, — — — — — — — and — — — —.

7. Basic amino acids are — — — — — — — — — and — — — — —.

8. Acidic amino acids are — — — — — — — — — — and — — — — — —.

9. Heterocyclic amino acids are — — — —, — — — — — — — and — — — — — — — — — — —.

10. The non-protein group in conjugated protein is called — — — — — —.

11. In glycoprotein the prosthetic group is — — — — — — — — — — —.

12. In chromoprotein the prosthetic group is — — — — — — — — —.

13. The most commonly used non-protein nitrogenous compounds are — — — — — and — — — — — — —.

14. The pH of the stomach for efficient protein digestion should be — — — — —.

15. The pancreatic enzymes namely — — — — —, — — — — — and — — — — — attack. the partial break down product of protein in duodenum.

16. In stomach, protein is attacked by enzymes namely — — — — — and — — — — — —.

17. Proteins are proteolyse into — — — — — — and — — — — — in rumen.

18. Excess of ammonia produced in rumen is carried to liver and converted into — — — — — — —.

19. The optimum level of ammonia in rumen is — — — — — — —.

20. Toxic level of ammonia in rumen liquor is — — — — — — — —.

21. Toxic level of ammonia in blood is — — — — — — — — — —.

22. — — — — — — — — ammonia concentration in blood is fatal.

23. Bureau of Indian Standards (BIS) recommended — — — — — urea in concentrate mixture.

24. The process of separation of nitrogen from an amino acid in the form of ammonia is called — — — — — — — —.

25. A process by which one amino acid results in the formation of another amino acid is called — — — — — — — —.

26. In transamination reaction pyruric acid is converted into — — — — — —. Whereas Asparatic acid is converted into — — — — — — —.

27. The end product of protein metabolism in birds is — — — — — —.

28. The two important reactions of protein metabolism are — — — — and — — —.

29. Urea is — — — percent degradable in rumen whereas fish meal degradability is — — — — — — —.

30. Acid detergent insoluble nitrogen (ADIN) is also called — — — — — —.

31. — — — — — — — — is the first limiting amino acids.

32. The disease of protein malnutrition of the young one is — — — — — — —.

33. — — — — — gram anhydrous sodium sulfate is added per gram of urea.

34. Urea is dificient in — — — — — — containing amino acids.

35. Urea has nitrogen content — — — — — gram/kg while Biuret has — — — — gram/kg.

36. Urea has crude protein content — — — — — — gram/kg while Biuret has — — — — — gram /kg.

37. Biuret is non-toxic at — — — — levels in comparison to urea, when added in ruminant feeds.

38. — — — — — — — — gave clear evidence that urea can utilized as protien source and needs for growth to ruminants.

39. To avoid ammonia toxicity not more than — — — — of dietary nitrogen should be provided as urea.

40. Urea does not provide the source of — — — — — — — —, — — — — — and — — — — —.

41. Arginine is breakdown into — — — — — — — and — — — — — — by the action of   arginase enzyme.

42. Rumen fluid has pronounced — — — — — — — — — activity which rapidly hydrolyzed   urea to ammonia and carbon dioxide.

43. Sugar present in DNA and RNA are — — — — — — — — — and — — — — — — — — — — — — —.

44. The basic protein present in cell nucleus and associated with DNA is referred as — — — — — — — — — —.

45. Positively charged amino acids are — — — — — — — — — , —
    — — — — — — — — — and — — — — — — —-

46. Phenyl alanine and tyrosine are — — — — — — — — — amino
    acids while Histidine   and tryptophane are — — — — —
    — — — — — amino acids.

Q.2. Explain the following:

1. NPN substance utilization in goat.
2. Digestion and absorption of protein in swine.
3. Digestion and absorption of protein and non-protein nitrogenous compound in cattle.
4. Protein metabolism in horse.
5. Transamination, deamination, amino acid toxicity, amino acid imbalance and antagonism, protein deficiency symptoms.
6. Factor affecting protein utilization in ruminants.
7. Urea feeding in ruminants.
8. Utilization of amino acids.
9. General function of protein.

Q.3. Differentiate the following:

1. Essential amino acid and non-essential amino acids.
2. Dispensable amino acid and non-dispensable amino acid.
3. Deamination and Transamination reactions.
4. Acidic amino acids and Basic amino acids.
5. Aromatic amino acids and aliphatic amino acid.
6. Fibrous protein and globular protein.
7. Conjugated protein and derived protein.

Chapter 6

The Lipids in Animal Nutrition

Plant and animal contain a group of substances, insoluble in water but soluble in ether, chloroform and benzene which are referred to as lipids. They act as electron carriers in enzymatic reactions, as component of biological membranes and as stores of energy. Fat contains 77, 12 and 11 percent carbon, hydrogen and oxygen, respectively. Certain compound lipids contain nitrogen and phosphorus also. The animal body contains 17 to 26 percent fat, which is stored around the walls of the intestine and kidney, fat depot under the skin and adipose tissues of the body. In addition to this, in small amount it is found in muscles and other parts of the body.

Function of fats:

1. The main function of fats is to supply energy to the animal body. One gram of fat after complete oxidation produces 9.3 Kcal heat. Fats are reserved source of energy to the animal body.

2. After hydrolysis, fats are converted into fatty acid and glycerol, so they provide essential fatty acids (linoleic, arachidonic and linolenic)· to the body.

3. It is an essential component of milk.

4. It helps in the absorption of calcium and phosphorus in the body.

5. Certain fat soluble vitamin such as vitamin, A,D,E, and K are absorbed in the blood in presence of fat.

6. It is an essential constituent of the body protoplasm.

7.   Phospholipids are the essential constituent of cell wall and play an important role in cell nutrition.
8.   It helps in temperature regulation & insulation for the vital organ, protecting them from shock.
9.   It is required for the lubrication of joints.
10. Fats are important nutrient of nervous metabolism.
11. It delays the sensation of hunger, as it requires a longer period of time to pass through the stomach than carbohydrate and protein.
12. Polyunsaturated F.A. particularly arachidonic acid, are the precursor of highly active prostaglandins.

Classification of Lipids:

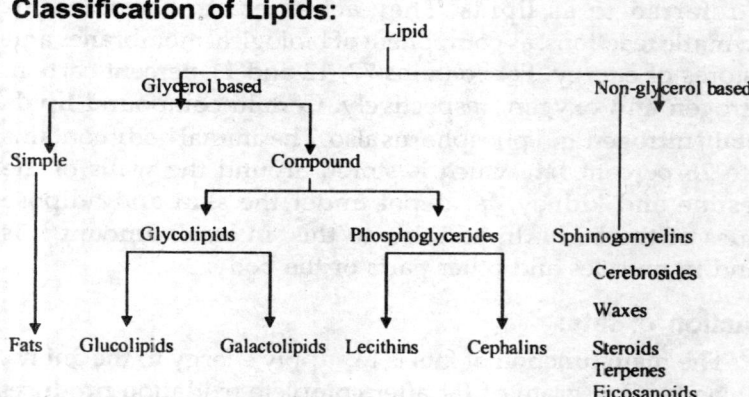

Fatty Acids: Fatty acids are long chain organic acids having usually from 4 to 30 carbon atoms, they have a single carboxyl group and a long non-polar hydrocarbon tail which gives most lipids their hydrophobic and oily or greasy nature. The chain may be saturated (containing only single bonds) or unsaturated (containing one or more double bonds).

Saturated Fatty Acids:

Trivial name	No. of C-atoms	Systemic name
Acetic acid	2	Ethanoic acid
Propionic acid	3	Propionic acid
Butyric acid	4	Butanoic acid

Caproic acid	6	Hexanoic acid
Caprylic acid	8	Octanoic acid
Capric acid	10	Decanoic acid
Lauric acid	12	Dodecanoic acid
Myristic acid	14	Tetra decanoic acid
Palmitic acid	16	Hexadecanoic acid
Stearic acid	18	Octa decanoic acid
Unsaturated Fatty Acid:		
Palmitoleic acid	(16-C):1	9 hexa decenoic acid
Oleic acid	(18-C) : 1	9 octa decenoic acid
Linoleic acid	(18-C) : 2	9,12 Octa decadienoic acid
Linolenic acid	(18-C) : 3	9,12,15 Octadecatrienoic acid
Arachidonic acid	(20-C) : 4	5,8,11,14 Icosa tetra enoic acid

Simple lipids: They are esters of fatty acid with trihydric alcohol glycerol. The most abundant are the fats and the less abundants are waxes.

Fats and Oils: Both have the same general structure and chemical properties but different physical characteristics. The melting point of the oils is such that at ordinary room temperature they are liquid. Chemically fats are ester of fatty acid with glycerol. In nature three fatty acid molecules combined with one glycerol molecule with release of three molecules of water.

$$CH_2OH \qquad\qquad CH_2.O.CO.R$$
$$|\qquad\qquad\qquad\qquad |$$
$$CHOH \; + \; 3 \, R.COOH \longrightarrow CH.O.CO.R \qquad + 3 \, H_2O$$
$$|\qquad\qquad\qquad\qquad |$$
$$CH_2 \, OH \qquad\qquad\qquad CH_2 \, O.CO.R$$

Glycerol   fatty acid   Triacylglycerol

Triglycerides differ in type according to the nature and position of the fatty acid residues. Those with three residues of the same fatty acid are termed simple triglycerides. When more than one fatty acids are esterfied with glycerol then a mixed triglycerides are formed.

$$CH_2. O.CO.R_1$$
$$|$$
$$CH.O.CO.R_2$$
$$|$$
$$CH_2.O.CO.R_3$$

Where, R_1, R_2 and R_3 represent the chains of different fatty acids.

Some of the fatty acids have one common property that they have a terminal carboxyl group and even number of carbon atoms, if derived from naturally occurring fat. The unsaturated fatty acids contain from one to many double bonds. Their physical properties are different from the saturated acids as they have lower melting points and are chemically more reactive.

Essential fatty acids: Three fatty acid viz. linoleic, linolenic and arachidonic acids are considered to be essential for farm animals. Either one of linoleic or arachidonic acid is capable of preventing the skin dermatitis caused by the deficiency of these acids in the chicks, pigs, calves and goats. Ruminant taking forages and grasses gets considerable quantities of linoleic acid. Hydrogenation of linoleic acid in the rumen will make available of more quantities of linolenic acid. Therefore, they are less likely to be affected by the deficiency of these acids.

Chemical properties of the fats:

Hydrolysis: Fats are hydrolysed to glycerol and fatty acid by the enzymes (lipases) and by alkali in the presence of water. Such a hydrolysis is known as saponification. The fats may be readily decomposed into glycerol and salt of the constituent fatty acid (soap) by boiling with strong bases such as sodium or potassium hydroxide.

Stearin + Potassium hydroxide = Potassium stearate (a soap) + Glycerol

Saponification number: The saponification number is defined as the milligrams of potassium hydroxide required to saponify 1 gram of fat. The saponification number of fat indicates the average molecular size of fatty acids.

Hydrogenation: The unsaturated glycerides of fat may be hydrogenated by treatment with hydrogen in the presence of nickel catalyst to form cooking fats. Oleic acid is hydrogenated to stearic acid.

Halogenation: Chlorine, bromine and iodine may be added to the double bonds of unsaturated glycerides in fats. It gives information about the number of unsaturated bond present in fats.

Iodine number: This is defined as the percent of iodine absorbed by the fat or the grams of iodine absorbed by 100 grams of fat.

Acetylation: The glycerides of fats containing hydroxylated fatty acids react with acetic anhydride and other acylating agents to form the corresponding esters.

Acetyl number: The acetyl number is defined as the milligram of KOH required to combine with the acetic acid liberated by the saponification of one gram of acetylated fat. Castor oil contain sufficient amount of hydroxylated acid to give a high acetyl number (146-150) whereas, butter has acetyl number of 1.9 to 8.6 indicating the presence of very small amount of hydroxylated acid.

Acid number: It is the milligrams of KOH required to neutralize the free fatty acids present in 1 gram of fat.

Reichert- Meissl number (R.M. Value): It is defined as the number of me. of decinormal alkali required to neutralize the steam volatile fatty acid from 5 g of fat.

Polenske Number: It is the number of milliliters of 0.1 N KOH required to neutralize the insoluble fatty acids obtained from 5 gram of fat.

Oxidation of unsaturated glycerides of fat: Oxidation of unsaturated bonds in the glycerides of fat absorbs oxygen and form products, which polymerize to produce insoluble hard films. Such oils are used in the production of paints and varnishes. The oxidation of unsaturated fatty acids takes place at the carbon atoms adjacent to the double bond to form hydroperoxides. The break down of hydroperoxides yields free radicals, which then attacked other fatty acids, and so more free radicals are produced and the process of oxidation increases exponentially. The products of oxidation include short chain fatty acids, fatty acid polymers, aldehydes, ketones, epoxides and hydrocarbons. Oxidation of saturated fatty acids results in the development of a sweet, heavy taste and smell commonly known as ketonic rancidity.

Rancidity of fat: When unsaturated fats or butter are stored they become rancid. It is of two types.

Hydrolytic rancidity: It is caused by the micro-organism in the fat in which short chain fatty acids are hydrolysed into malodourous fatty acids. But nutritive value of fat in hydrolytic rancidity remains same.

Oxidative rancidity: Oils containing highly unsaturated F.A. are spontaneously oxidized into short chain F.A. (C_4 to C_{10}) and aldehydes by atmospheric oxygen at ordinary temperature. This rancidity develops in the fat by autooxidation. It is more common in unsaturated fatty acids. Due to oxidation, hydroperoxides are broken down to aldehyde and ketone, which have offensive taste and smell. As the structure is altered, the nutritive value of fat is reduced in this type of rancidity. The vitamin E and hydroxyquinone are antioxidants which are used to prevent rancidity or oxidation of fat oxidative rancidity is observed more frequently in animal fats than in vegetable fats. This is due to the presence of natural antioxidants eg. Tocopherol, phenols, napthols which checks autooxidation. Synthetic anti oxidants such as Nordihdroguia retic acid (NDGA) & Tertiary butyl hydroxy anisole (BHA) are also used for preventing oxidative rancidity.

Oxidative rancidity:

$$R - CH_2 - CH = CH - CH_2 - R \quad + \quad O_2 \longrightarrow$$

$$R - \underset{\underset{\displaystyle H}{\overset{\displaystyle O}{\underset{|}{O}}}}{CH} - CH = CH - CH_2 - R$$

O   Hydroperoxide

$$R - \underset{O^0}{\underset{|}{CH}} - CH = CH - CH_2 - R + OH^0$$

O^0 Free radicals

$$R^0 + O_2 \longrightarrow RO_2{}^0$$

$$RO_2{}^0 + RH \longrightarrow R^0 + ROOH$$

$$R^0 + R^0 \longrightarrow R\text{-}R$$

Autocatalytic oxidation of fatty acids

Waxes: Waxes are defined as the esters of higher fatty acids and of higher monohydroxy alcohol. They are found in numerous reactions in plants, animals and microorganism where they form a protective covering and are present in oily secretion.

Beeswax: This insect wax is a complex mixture of ester, some fatty acids, alcohols and hydroxarbons. It contains mainly the myricyl palmitate as the ester.

Lanolin or wool fat: This material forms a protective coating over the wool fibres and is a wax rather than fat. Lanolin has the properties of taking up much water without dissolving, which make it a valuable as a medium in the preparation of ointments, cosmetics and candles.

Compound lipids:

(A) Phospholipids (Phosphatides):

These are lipids, which contain phosphorus, the latter being present as esterified phosphoric acid. Among the many vital functions, regulation of plant and animal cell permeability, participation in the transport and metabolism of synthesized and dietary fats and role in blood coagulations are important.

$$\begin{array}{lcl}
CH_2OH & & CH_2OCOR_1 \\
| & & | \\
CHOH + R_1\,COOH + R_2\,COOH + H_3PO_4 & \longrightarrow & CHOCOR_2 \\
| & & |\quad\; O \\
 & & \quad\;\;\; \| \\
CH_2OH & & CH_2O{-}P{-}OH \\
 & & \quad\;\;\; | \\
\text{Glycerol} & & \quad\;\;\; OH \\
 & & \text{Phosphatidic acid}
\end{array}$$

1. Phosphoglycerdes:

(a) Lecithins: Like fats, lecithins are ester of glycerol. Two of the alcohol groups are esterified with fatty acid, but the third is estrified with phosphoric acid, which is inturn esterified by the nitrogenous base choline. A typical example would have the formula:

$$\begin{array}{lcl}
 & & CH_2\,O.CO.\,C_{15}\,H_{31} \\
\quad\quad\quad\quad OH & & | \\
\text{Phosphatidic acid} + CH_2CH_2\,N^+\,(CH_3)_3 & \longrightarrow & CH.P.CO.C_{17}\,H_{33} \\
\quad\quad\quad\quad \text{Choline} & & | \\
 & & CH_2.O.PO^-_3.CH_2.CH_2.\,N^+\,(CH_3)_3
\end{array}$$

The chief fatty acid present are palmitic, stearic, arachidic and oleic. Acids below lauric are not found in the lecithins.

(b) ***Cephalin:*** Cephalin differs from the lecithins in having ethanolamine instead of choline and is correctly termed as phosphatidyl enthanolamine. Cephalin has the following formula:

$$\begin{array}{lcl}
 & & CH_2.O.CO.R \\
\text{Phosphatidic acid} + OH\,CH_2\,CH_2\,NH_2 & \longrightarrow & | \\
\quad\quad\quad\quad \text{Ethanolamine} & & CH.O.CO.R \\
 & & | \\
 & & CH_2.O.PO^-_3.CH_2CH_2.\,NH_2
\end{array}$$

Cephalin usually contains stearic, oleic, linolenic and arachidonic acid.

(c) Phosphatidyl serine: They differ from lecithins in having serine as their nitrogenous base which is phosphatidyl serine having formula:

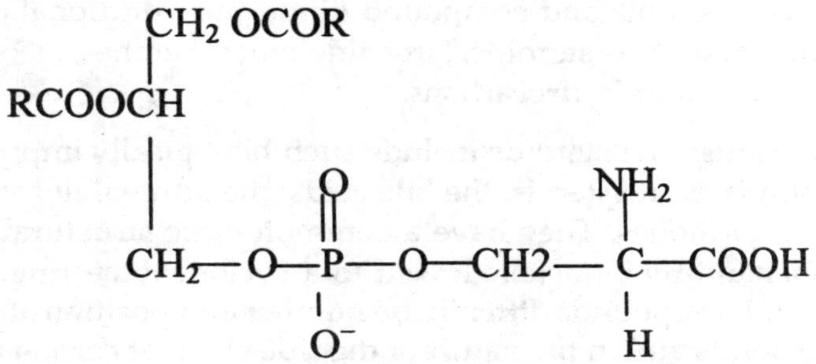

$$CH_2\ OCOR$$

$$RCOOCH$$

$$CH_2-O-\overset{\overset{O}{\|}}{P}-O-CH2-\overset{\overset{NH_2}{|}}{C}-COOH$$

$$O^-\qquad\qquad H$$

(d) Plasmogens: Some phosphoglycerides contain enol form of a long-chain aldehyde connected by ether linkage and replacing one fatty acid found in lecthins and cephalins.

2. Phophoinositides: These compounds on hydrolysis yield glycerol, fatty acid, inositol and phosphate. Inositol is a vitamin. Two different types of phosphoinositides have been described by the inositol derivatives yielded upon hydrolysis. Monophosphoinositide found in heart, liver, soyabean and wheat germ and diphosphoinositide found in brain.

3. Phosphosphinosides (sphingomyelins): These compounds are found in nervous tissue and differ from phosphoglycerides in the nature of nitrogenous base components and lack of glycerol. They are madeup of fatty acids, phosphoric acid, choline and sphigosine. The general formula of sphingomyelins is given below:

$$CH_3\ (CH_2)_{12}.\ CH{:}CH.\ CHOH.\ CH.\ CH_2\ O.PO^-{}_3.\ CH_2.\ CH_2.\ N^+\ (CH_3)_3$$

$$|$$

$$NH.CO.R$$

(B) Glycolipids (Glycosphigosides or cerbrosides):

The glycolipids are compounds occurring most commonly in nerve tissues. They consist of fatty acid residue, usually of high molecular weight, linked to the amino group of sphingosine which is linked via its terminal alcohol group to a molecule of hexose **sugar**; this is most frequently galactose and less often glucose.

Derived lipids: Derived lipids on hydrolysis give the products of simple and compound lipids and additional other compounds such as steroids, fatty aldehydes, ketones, alcohols, essential oils and hydrocarbons.

Steroids: The steroids include such biologically important compounds as the sterols, the bile acids, the adrenal hormones and sex hormones. They have a common basic structural unit of a phenanthrene nucleus linked to a cyclopentane ring. The individual compounds differ in the number and position of their double bonds and in the nature of the side chain at carbon atom 17.

Sterols: These have 8 to 10 carbon atoms in the side chain, and an alcohol group at carbon atom 3. They may be classified into:

1.	The phytosterol of plant origin
2.	The mycosterol of fungal origin
3.	The Zoosterols of animal origin.

Cholesterol: Cholesterol is zoosterol which is quantitatively an important constituent of the brain. It occurs in smaller amounts in all animal cells and it can be synthesized in the body, but, inspite of this wide distribution and apparent importance little is known of its actual function. The thickening is due to deposition of cholesterol inside the arterial walls.

7-Dehydrocholesterol: Which is derived from cholesterol is an important precursor of vitamin D_3, which is produced when the sterol is exposed to ultraviolet light.

Ergosterol: It is a phytosterol widely distributed in brown algae, bacteria and higher plants. It is important as the precursor of ergocalciferol or vitamin D_2

Bile acids: The bile acids have a five carbon side chain at carbon 17 terminating in a carboxyl group which is bound by an amide linkage to glycine or taurine. The bile acids are important in the duodenum where they aid the emulsification of fats and the activation of lipase.

Steroid Hormones: These include male sex hormone (androgens), and female sex hormones (oestrogen and progesterone) as well as cortisol, aldosterone and corticosterone which are produced by the adrenal cortex.

Essential oils: Many terpenes found in plants have strong characteristic odours and flavours and are components of essential oils such as lemon or camphor oil. The word essential is used here to indicate the occurrence of the oils in essences and not to imply that the animals require them. Among the many important plant terpenes are the phytol moiety of chlorophyll, the carotenoid pigments and the vitamin A, E, and K. In animal some of the co-enzymes are terpenes.

Digestion and absorption of lipid in non-ruminants: Fat and cholesterol are not miscible with water whereas, phospholipids are much more miscible. Lipid digestion and absorption require arranging the lipid in a form that is water miscible to cross the microvilli of the small intestine, which are covered with aquous layer.

Peristaltic movement of stomach and duodenum made it as a coarse emulsion. The pancreatic lipase and colipase in the presence of bile hydrolyze the triglyceride droplets into fatty acids and monoglycerides and reduce the lipid to a finer and finer emulsion. 2-monoglyceride, which has a polar (glycerol) and non-polar (fatty acid) end, is an excellent emulsifying agent. The bile, free fatty acids and monoglyceride become oriented into a mixed micelle containing a lipid core and a polar exterior. Micelles are tiny particles formed by the combination of bile salts with the free fatty acids and monoglycerides produced during digestion.

The micelle migrates to the brush border where it is disrupted. Most of the bile is absorbed into the mucosa and the remaining bile in the lumen moves down the intestine and absorbed and recirculated through the liver.

Most of the triglycerides are absorbed upto the mid jejunum. With in the mucosa, the fatty acids and monoglycerides are resynthesized into triglycerides, combined with cholesterol and phospholipid encased in a thin layer of protein and secreted into the central lacteal of the villus as either chylomicron or very low density lipoprotein (VLDL) particles. Chylomicron is responsible for transportation of dietary fat to various tissues in the body. The central lacteal drains into the lymph vessels and enters the general blood circulation via the thoracic duct at the right atrium. The hydrolysis and resynthesis of triglycerides during the process of digestion and absorption produces similar but not identical triglyceride molecules in the lymph. The absorption rate is more, if dietary lipid contains

*1. Shorter chain length fatty acids

*2. More unsaturated fatty acids

*3. As triglycerides rather than free fatty acids.

Digestion and absorption of lipid in ruminants: The ruminant diet consists of a high proportion of unsaturated fatty acids found in galactolipids of forage and in the triglycerides of the cereal grains. The rumen microbial population hydrolyzes the triglyceride and galactolipid, releasing free fatty acids (FFA) and fermented the glycerol and galactose into volatile fatty acids. The process of hydrogenation saturates the unsaturated fatty acids. The bacteria and protozoa are also capable of synthesizing a number of odd chain fatty acids from propionate and branched chain fatty acids from the carbon skeltons of the amino acids valine, leucine and isoleucine. Lipid is present in the form of thin layer of free fatty acids on the surface of the feed particles in duodenum. A little triglyceride is available to be converted to monoglyceride in duodenum and upper jejunum because of acidic content of duodenum and upper jejunum. So active micelle formation of the fatty acids does not occur in the upper tract under the influence of bile salts and lecithin.

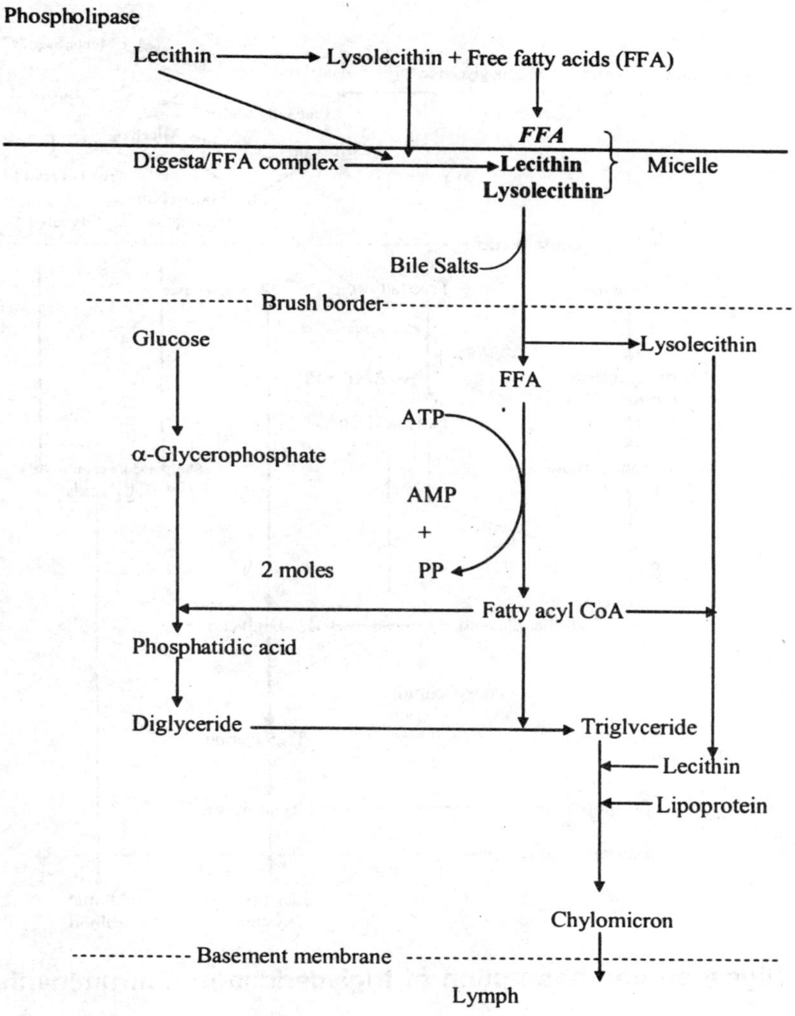

Phospholipase

Lecithin ⟶ Lysolecithin + Free fatty acids (FFA)

FFA

Digesta/FFA complex ⟶ **Lecithin** } Micelle
Lysolecithin

Bile Salts

------------------ Brush border-------------------------------------

Glucose ⟶ Lysolecithin

FFA

ATP

α-Glycerophosphate

AMP

+

2 moles   PP ⟵

Fatty acyl CoA ⟶

Phosphatidic acid

Diglyceride ⟶ Triglvceride

⟵ Lecithin

⟵ Lipoprotein

Chylomicron

------------- Basement membrane -------------------------------------

Lymph

Absorption of dietary fat in the small intestine of ruminants.

In lower three quarter of the jejunum the pancreatic phospholipase hydrolyze lecithin into a fatty acid and lysolecithin, which further enhances micelle formation. So absorption of lipid takes place in lower two third of jejunum.

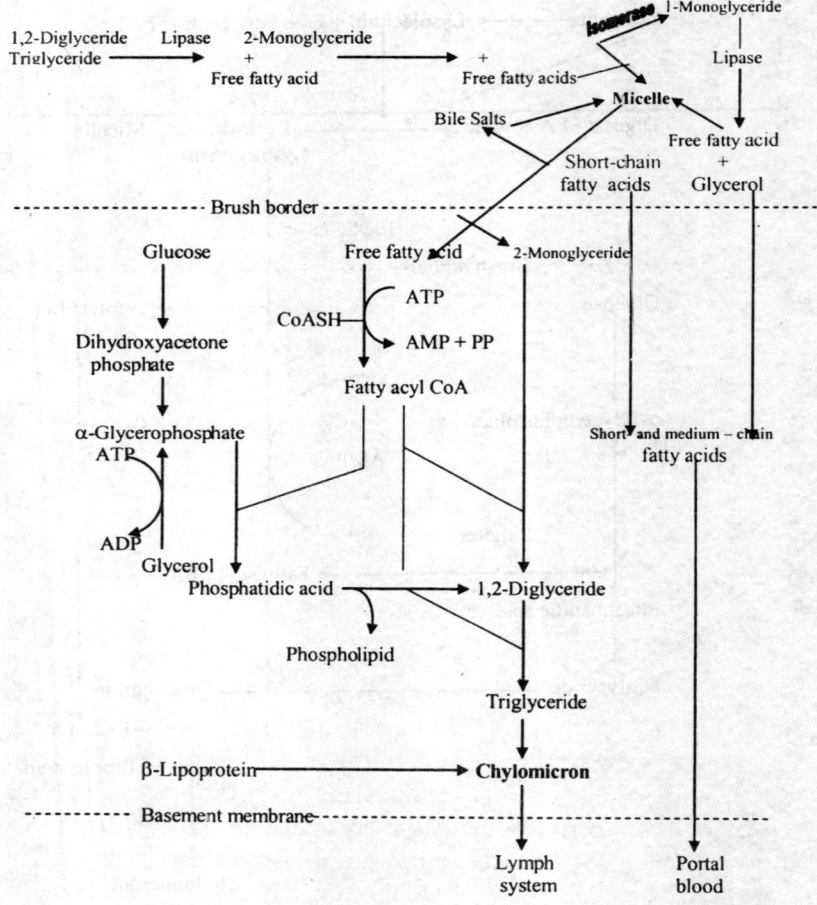

Digestion and absorption of triglycerides in nonruminants

Metabolism of lipids: The digestion of lipids produces glycerol and fatty acids, which are metabolised and produce energy.

Metabolism of glycerol: Glycerol is glycogenic in nature and converted into dihydroxy acetone phsophate.

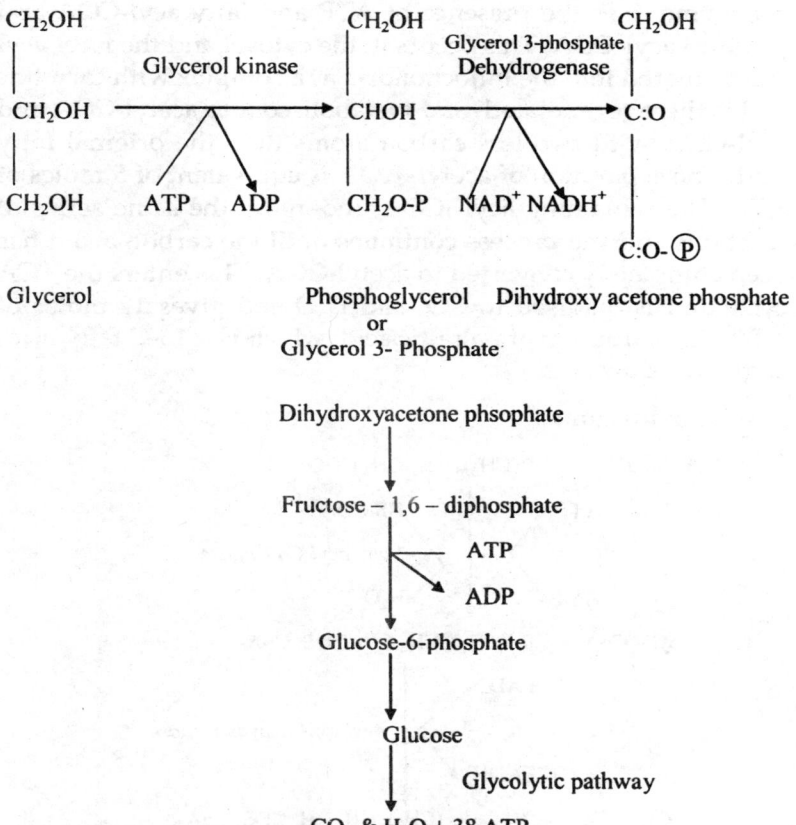

Conversion of 2-mole glycerol to dihydroxyaceton phosphate produces 6 moles of ATP and utilizes 2 mole of ATP, whereas conversion of 2 moles of dihydroxyacetone phosphate to one mole of glucose and glucose metabolism via glycolytic pathway produces 38 moles of ATP. So a net

$$\frac{38+6-2}{2} = 21$$ moles of ATP are produced per mole of glycerol.

Metabolism of fatty acids: The fatty acid provides the major part of the energy derived from the fat. The fatty acid is metabolised by β-oxidation mechanism, which shortened the carbon chain by removing two carbon atoms at a time. The first stage of this mechanism is the reaction of the fatty acid with

99

coenzyme A in the presence of ATP and fatty acyl-COA and produce acyl-COA. This occurs in the cytosol and the fatty acyl-COA entered into the mitochondria as a complex with carnitine and is there regenerated- and metabolised into acetyl-COA and acyl-COA with two less carbon atoms than the original fatty acid. The separation of acetyl- COA is equivalent of 5 moles of ATP. The remaining acyl- COA undergoes the same series of reactions and the process continues until the carbon chain has been completely converted to acetyl-COA. This enters the TCA cycle and is oxidised to CO_2 and H_2O and gives 12 moles of ATP. The oxidation of palmitic acid, which is a 16-C fatty acid, is given below:

β- oxidation:

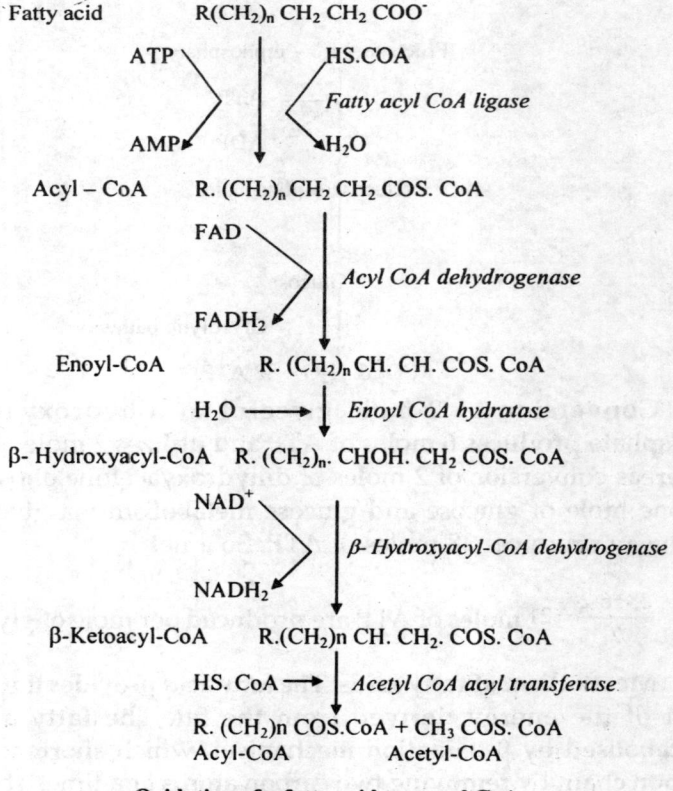

Oxidation of a fatty acid to acetyl CoA

Energy production from palmitic acid:

1 Mole palmitic acid to palmitoyl-COA = - 2 ATP

1 Mole palmitoyl- COA to 8 moles acetyl – COA = + 35 ATP

8 Moles acetyl- COA to CO_2 and H_2O = + 96 ATP

Net gain of ATP per mole of palmitic acid = 129. Similarly stearic acid (18-C) produces a net gain of 146 ATP and archidic acid (20-C) produces a net gain of 163 ATP per mole of archidic acid.

Q.1. Fill in the blanks with appropriate words.

1. Fat contains _____ percent carbon.

2. _____, _____ and _____ are essential fatty acids.

3. _____ and _____ are simple lipids.

4. When more than one fatty acids are esterifed with glycerol then a _____ are formed.

5. Fatty acids containing more than one double bonds are called _____.

6. Milligram of potassium hydroxide required to saponity 1 gram of fat is called _____.

7. The process of hydrolysis of fats in which soaps are formed is known as _____.

8. Iodine number is the amount of iodine absorbed by _____ grams of fat.

9. Acetyl number is milligram of _____ required combining with the acetic acid liberated by the saponification of one gram of acetylated fat.

10. _____ type of rancidity affect the nutritive value of fat.

11. _____ type of rancidity does not affect the nutritive value of fat.

12. The number of ml. of decinormal alkali required to neutralize the steam volatile fatty acid from 5 g of fat is called _____.

13. Lecithin contains a nitrogenous base called _____.

14. Cephalin differs from the lecithin in having _____ group instead of choline.

15. Most of the triglycerides are absorbed at _____ in GIT.
16. The digestion of lipid produces _____ and _____.
17. Metabolism of one mole of glycerol produces _____ ATP.
18. Fatty acids are metabolised by _____ process.
19. The separation of acetyl COA from fatty acids yields _____ moles of ATP.
20. Acetyl COA produced from fatty acids in metabolised are produce _____ moles of ATP.
21. A net gain of _____ moles of ATP is produced by 1 mole palmitic acid metabolism.
22. Complete metabolism of steraric acid produces _____. Moles of ATP.
23. Complete metabolism of 1 mole of arachidonic acid produces _____ moles of ATP.
24. Fatty acid is metabolized by ————————————— which shortened two carbon atoms at a time.
25. Chylomicron is responsible for transportation of ———— ——————————————to various tissues in the body.

Q.2. Explain the following:
1. Explain the digestion and absorbtion of lipids in ruminants.
2. Explain the digestion and absorption of lipids in non-ruminants.
3. How the glucerol is metabolised in the body?
4. Explain the metabolism of fatty acids by β-oxidation mechanism.
5. How much ATP are produced from metabolism of 1 mole of palmitic acid, steraric acid and archidic acid each and How?
6. Define the terms:

Saponification number, Iodine number, Acetyl number, Reichert- Meissl number, Hydrolytic and oxidative rancidity in fat, Saponification and acetylation of fats.

Chapter 7

The Minerals in Animal Nutrition

The periodic system lists 104 elements. There are about 40 mineral elements that occur in measurable amount in nature in the plants and animals tissues. Minerals are generally classified into two categories.

1.   **Macro elements (Major elements):** The minerals, which are required in relatively large amount and in most of cases they are used in the synthesis of structural tissues. Their concertration is expressed in term of percentage. The important major elements are calcium, phosphorus, magnesium, sodium, potassium, chlorine and sulphur.

2.   **Micro elements (Minor elements or trace elements):** These minerals required in trace amounts and usually function as activators or as a component of enzyme system. The concentration of trace elements is expressed in terms of part per million (PPM) since their concentration is very low in the plants and body. The important trace elements are iron, copper, iodine, cobalt, zinc, manganese, fluorine, selenium, molybdenum, chromium, nickel, silicon, tin and vanadium and play a functional role in animal physiology.

Essential mineral elements: These are those minerals, which have been proved to have a metabolic role in the animal body.

Non-essential mineral elements: Most of mineral elements are simply component of animal tissues since they are present in the diet and are considered to be non-essential, as they do not play any essential metabolic role in the plant or animal body.

General Function of Minerals: The functions of minerals in animal nutrition are inter-related. However, a few of the general functions are given as:

1. As a constituent of skeletal structure:

2. In regulating acid-base equilibrium.

3. They are helpful in maintaining the colloridal state of body matter and regulating some of the physical properties of colloidal systems like viscosity, diffusion and osmotic pressure.

4. They act as a component or an activator of enzymes and or other biological systems.

MACRO-ELEMENTS (MAJOR ELEMENTS): All the macrominerals are discussed here reference to their function, metabolism, deficiency symptoms and sources of these minerals.

1. Calcium: Calcium and phosphorus serve as the major structural elements of skeletal tissue, with more than 99 per cent of the total body calcium being found in the bone and teeth. The normal level of blood calcium in animals ranges from 9 to 11 mg per 100 ml of serum. The cell contains negligible amounts. From 45-50 per cent of the plasma calcium is in the soluble, ionized form, while 40-45 per cent is bound with protein, primarily albumin and other plasma protein. The remaining 5 per cent is complexed with non-ionized inorganic elements depending on blood pH. The plasma of laying hens contains 30 to 40 mg calcium per 100 ml of blood.

Factors affecting the level of blood calcium:

1. **The absolute levels of calcium and phosphorus and the calcium phosphorus ratio of food:** A low intake of either element over long periods of time leads to decreased blood calcium level. A Ca: P ratio of 1:1 to 2:1 is usually recommended.

2. **Fat content in the diet:** Impaired digestion and absorption of fat causes impaired absorption of calcium because calcium form soaps which are insoluble.

3. **Phytic acid and oxalate:** Oxalates in certain foods precipi-

tate calcium in the intestine as the insoluble calcium oxalates formed insoluble salt with calcium and makes it insoluble.

4. **Acidity relation:** Acidic medium in intestine favour calcium absorption.

5. **Protein in the diet:** Calcium salts are much more soluble in amino acid than water. High protein level increases the absorption of calcium.

6. **Vitamin D in the diet:** Vitamin D provides acidic medium in the intestine causing more calcium absorption.

7. **Parathyroid hormones:** Parathyroid hormones regulate calcium level in the plasma.

8. **Kidney threshold:** In a normal adult any extra calcium absorded from the kidney is readily excreted in the urine.

9. **Sex hormone:** Low level of oestrogen hormone causes poor absorbtion of calcium.

Function of calcium: Calcium is essential for skeletal formation, normal blood clotting, rhythmic heart action, neuromuscular excitability, enzyme activation and permeablity of membranes and acid base balance of body fluid and also in curdling of milk. A number of enzymes including lipase, succinic dehydrogenase, adenosinetriphophataseand certain proteolytic enzymes are activated by calcium.

Absorption of calcium: The main site of calcium absorption is the small intestine specially the proximal portion of the duodenum. The percentage of absorption of calcium decreases with age, high F intakes, and high ca intakes or low vitamin D intakes. The major route of excretion for calcium is through faeces.

Requirement of calcium	(% of dry matter infeed
Lactating cows	0.43-0.60%
Sheep	0.21-0.52%
Goat	0.21-0.52%
Poultry	0.80-1.20%

Deficiency symptoms:

1. **Ricket:** This symptoms occure in young growing animals. The symptoms of rickets are misshapen bones, enlargement of joints, lameness and stiffiness. This condition is called Ricketic rosary. Calcification of normal bone does not take place.

2. **Osteomalacia:** In the adult animals, calcium deficiency results in osteomalacia. In osteomalacia the bones become weak, porous and soft. Continuous mobilization of calcium from the bones for the higher demand with a low intake is responsible for this condition.

3. **Osteoporosis:** This is characterized by a decreased bone mass. It is due to bone resorption being greater than bone formation. It is prominent in aging, and related to gonadal hormone deficiency.

4. **Milk fever (parturient paresis; calcium tetany):** Shortly after parturition, high yielding cows may suffer from milk fever. The serum calcium goes down with the result that there are muscular spasms and in extreme cases paralysis. There may be breeding difficulties in pregnant animals and the calves born may be dead or very weak.

5. In laying hens deficiency of calcium results in improper development of the egg-shell which is either not fully formed or easily breakable. The deficiency causes soft bones and beak, curved legs and low egg production.

Source of calcium: Milk and green leafy crops, especially legumes, are good sources of calcium; cereals and roots are poor sources. Animal by product containing bone, fish meal, meat cum bone meal are rich source of calcium. Dicalcium phosphate, calcium carbonate and calcium phosphate are also good source of calcium.

Calcium content of feed stuff:

Feed stuff	% Calcium
Barley	0.09
Maize	0.04
Wheat	0.05
Wheat bran	0.16
Soyabean meal	0.36
Cow milk	0.91
Spinach	1.00
Eggs	0.19
Bone meal	27.3
Dicalcium phosphate	23.1
Lime stone	33.8
Oyster shell	38.0
Legume forages	1.42
Grasses	0.37

2. Phosphorous: Major portion of phosphorus in the animal body is distributed in the bones. The content of inorganic phosphorus in the blood is 4 to 9 mg per 100 ml depending upon the species and age. Maintenance of inorganic phosphorus level in the blood is also governed by the same factors, which promote calcium and phosphorus assimilation. Whole blood contains about 35-40 mg phosphorus per 100 ml.

Functions of Phosphorus:

1. Phosphorus plays an important role in the formation of bones and teeth along with calcium. The amount of phosphorus present in these structure in about 80 per cent of the total.

2. It maintained the normal level of blood calcium and its proper activity.

3. It plays active role for the formation of phospholipid in the cells, nucleic acid, coenzyme, phosphoprotein and phospholipid.

4. It plays a vital role or in energy metabolism in the formation of sugar phosphate like adenosine di-phosphate (ADP) and triphosphates (ATP).

Deficiency symptoms:

1. **Rickets:** Deficiency of phosphorus causes ricket along with calcium imbalance in young animals.

2. **Osteomalacia:** The element causes osteomalacia in adult with deficiency of calcium.

3. **Pica (Depraved appetite):** Phosphorus deficiency causes a specific symptom in cattle called pica. The affected animals have abnormal appetites and chew woods, bone, rags and other foreign materials. The animals become very weak, if not treated, they may die due to weakness or due to secondary infections, which occur from eating decaying bones and other materials.

4. **Reproduction:** Low dietary intake of phosphorus has also been associated with poor fertility; dysfunction of ovaries causing inhibition, depression and irregularity of oestrus.

Requirements of phosphorus (% of dry matter in feed):

Dairy cows	0.31-0.40
Sheep / Goat	0.16-0.37
Poultry	0.32-0.50

Sources of Phosphorus: Animal products like fish meal, meat meal and bone meal are good sources of phosphorus. Cereal grains, wheat bran, rice bran, rice polishing, cake etc. are fairly good sources of phosphorus though poor source of calcium. Leguminous fodders like berseem and lucerne are poor sources of phosphorus. Most of the phosphorus present in the cereals and their by-products is in the form of phytates, which are the salt of phytic acid, a phosphoric acid derivative. Ruminants can utilize the phytate phosphorus due to rumen microbial activity.

Phosphorus content of feed stuffs:

Feed stuffs	Phosphorus (%)
Barley	0.47
Maize	0.31
Wheat	0.41

Wheat bran	1.32
Soyabean meal	0.75
Spinach	0.55
Cow milk	0.71
Egg	0.83
Bone meal	13.0
Dicalcium phosphate	18.7
Rock phosphate	18.0

3. Magnesium: About 70 percent of the total magnesium is found in the skeleton, the remainder being distributed in soft tissues and fluids. Blood serum contain 2 to 3 mg magnesium per 100 ml. Bone contains about 1.5 percent magnesium.

Function of Magnesium:

1. Magnesium plays important role in activating various enzymes such as phosphate transferases, decarboxylases and acyltransferases.

2. Magnesium is an activator of phosphates and takes an active part in the carbohydrate metabolism.

3. It also plays an important role in calcium and phosphorus metabolism for the formation of bone and teeth.

4. Magnesium also plays an important role for the neuromuscular activity of the body.

Absorption of magnesium: The rumen and reticulum is the major site of Mg absorption in ruminants. It is also absorbed from large intestine. Magnesium is excreted via faeces, urine and milk.

Requirement of magnesium	% of dry matter
Dairy cow	0.20
Sheep and goat	0.04-0.08

Deficiency symptoms:

1. Magnesium tetany in adult animals (Grass staggers, Grass tetany): It is also referred as lactation tetany or wheat pasture poisoning. There are other factors also which are responsible for gross staggers like hormonal disturbances and faulty interrelationship of calcium, phosphorus and magnesium. Clinical signs of tetany include appetite, increased excitability, profuse salivation and convulsions.

2. Hypomagnesimia in young calves: This has been reported in India when calves reared on milk diet without any other supplement for a prolonged period.

3. Neurological symptoms in rats: In the rats lowering of magnesium to 1.8 ppm resulted in hyper-irritability, convulsion and death. The blood picture showed normal calcium and phosphorus but magnesium content was reduced. In poultry magnesium deficiency causes neurological symptoms like rats.

Sources of Magnesium: Most of the commonly fed roughage and concentrates contain 0.1 percent. Bran, oil cakes and leguminous fodder are rich source of magnesium while milk and animal products are much poorer source.

Magnesium content of some feed stuffs:

Feed stuffs	Magnesium (mg/100gm)
Egg	11
Cow milk	12
Spinach	97
Corn	121
Peas	140
Wheat	165
Soybean	210

4. Sodium: It is an alkaline salt which forms about 93 percent alkali of blood serum. It is found in body fluids and muscles of the body. The total amount of sodium in the body is about 0.2 percent out of which upto 0.05 percent is deposited in bones.

Functions of Sodium:
1. Sodium salt is useful in the metabolism of water, protein, fat and carbohydrate.
2. It controls body fluid concentration, contraction of nerve and muscle fibres, body fluid pH, osmotic pressure and

help in maintaining neutrality among body tissues.

Absorption of sodium: Absorption of sodium takes place in rumen and upper small intestine. It is mainly excreted through urine with small amount is also excreted through faeces and perspiration.

Requirement of sodium	% of dry matter in feed
Sheep and goat	0.04-0.10
Poultry	0.11-0.14
Dry cow	0.18-0.20

Deficiency symptoms: The deficiency of sodium in the body of animals result in loss of appetite, general debility, stoppage of growth and development, fall of body temperature, neuromuscular disturbances and loss of milk production in lactating animals.

Feed stuff	Sodium (%)
Maize	0.03
Oat	0.13
Wheat	0.10
Soyabean	0.35
Wheat straw	0.12
Grasses	0.03
Wheat bran	0.14
Fish meal	1.06

Sources of sodium: The chief source of sodium is sodium cloride or common salt. Most of the feed and forages are poor source of sodium except the herbage which grown on alkaline soil for reclamation.

5. Potassium: Most of the potassium is found in the cells. Excess of this salt in the body interferes with the absorption and metabolism of magnesium.

Functions of Potassium:

1. Potassium is essential part along with sodium, chlorine and bicarbonate ions, in the osmotic pressure regulation of the body fluids and in the acid-base balance in the animals.

2. Potassium plays an important role in nerve and muscles excitability and activates certain enzymes.

Absorption of potassium: Potassium is absorbed mainly from the small intestine and to some extent in the large intestine. The majority of potassium excretion is in the urine and also via sweat and milk.

Deficiency symptoms:

1. Potassium deficiency result in slow growth, reduced feed and water intake, lowered feed efficiency, muscular weakness, nervous disorders, stiffness, emaciation, intracellular acidisis and degeneration of vital organs.

2. High intake of potassium may interfere with the absorption and metabolism of magnesium in the animals, which may be an important factor in the etiology of hypomagnesaemic tetany.

Sources of potassium: Outside the body potassium is available in pasture grasses. Milk also contains potassium. Inside the body it is found in muscles, plasma and blood cells.

6. Chlorine: It is found in skin, subcutaneous tissues and gastric juices. Out of the total amount present in the body 80-85 percent chloride is found in inorganic form while the rest 15 to 20 percent in organic form.

Functions of Chlorine:

1. This mineral is required for the formation of hydrochloric acid of the gastric juice.

2. In the form of sodium chloride it assists in the digestion of food.

3. Chlorine is associated with sodium and potassium in acid base relationship and osmotic regulation.

4. It also helps in cell nutrition, growth and reproduction among animals.

Absorption of chlorine: Chlorine is absorbed in combination with sodium. It is mainly absorbed from the upper small intestine. It is excreted through urine with small amount in faeces and perspiration.

Deficiency symptoms:

1. A dietary deficiency of chlorine may lead to an abnormal increase of the alkali reserve of the blood (alkalosis) caused by an excess of bicarbonate, since inadequate levels of chlorine in the body are party compensated for by increase in bicarbonate.

2. Deficiency of salt in diet leads to decreased appetite which result in poor growth rate and milk production.

3. Deficiency of salt in poultry leads to feather picking and canabalism.

Sources of chlorine: With the exception fish and meat meals, the chlorine content of most foods is comparatively low. The chlorine content of pasture grass varies from 3 to 25 g/kg dry matter. The main source of this element for most animals is common salt.

7. Sulphur: Most of the sulphur in the animal body occurs in proteins containing the amino acids cystine, cysteine and methionine. The two vitamins, biotin and thiamin and the hormone, insulin, also contain sulphur.

Functions of Sulphur:

1. Sulphur is an essential element for protein and vitamin synthesis. Wool is rich in cystine and contains about 4 percent of sulphur.

2. It combined with iron and used for the formation of heamoglobin in red blood cells.

3. It also useful in blood clotting and endocrine function.

4. It also maintained intra and extra cellular fluid and acid base balance.

Absorption of sulphur: Sulphur is absorbed in the rumen and small intestine. It can be recycled to the rumen with similarities to the recycling system for the urea-nitrogen system.

Deficiency symptoms:

1. Deficiency of sulphur in the body results in poor growth and development of the body, loss of weight, weakness,

lacrimation and metabolic activities of the body are also disturbed. Microbial protein synthesis is reduced and the animal shows sign of protein malnutrition. There is evidence that sodium sulphate can be by used ruman microorganisms more efficiently than elemental sulphur.

2. In sheep its deficiency causes production of the poor quality wool.

Sources of sulphur: All balanced rations, muscles, wings of the birds, horns, hairs, nails, bile juice, saliva, R.B.C, nervous system and hoof of the animals contain certain amount of sulphur.

Sulphur content in feed stuffs:

Feed stuffs	Sulphur (%)
Maize	0.15
Wheat	0.17
Soyabean	0.41
Alfalfa hay	0.16
Fish meal	0.11
Dried skim milk	0.08

TRACE ELEMENTS (MICRO ELEMENTS): Various trace minerals are discussed here. The average trace minerals content of various feeds and fodders are mentioned below:

Average traces mineral contents of feed stuffs:

Feed stuffs	Mg/kg air dry feed stuffs					
	Fe	Cu	Co	Mn	Zn	I
1. Cereals and leguminous crops						
a. Maize	36	5.0	0.02	5	22	0.30
b. Barley	48	6.4	0.08	15	22	0.25
c. Wheat	50	6.2	0.08	30	26	0.07
d. Soyabeans	125	17.0	0.10	31	35	0.20
2. Maize silage	196	7.0	0.08	42	32	0.06
3. Alfalfa hay	188	11.0	0.09	41	13.5	0.03
4. Wheat straw	120	3.4	0.03	32	67	0.30
5. Cotton seed cake	190	19.0	0.28	21	80	0.30
6. Wheat bran	90	11.0	0.80	119	95	0.09
7. Fish meal	340	7.5	0.80	19	103	2.50
8. Dried skim milk	9	0.7	0.07	2.2	45	0.03

1. Iron: The total amount of iron found in the body is 0.004 percent. Half of this amount remains in combination with R.B.C. in the form of heme associated with red colouring matter or haemoglobin. The remaining portion is found associated with myoglobin, enzyme cytochrome, peroxidase, catalase and other enzymes of the body; liver, spleen and kidney. As a respiratory enzyme it is present in all the tissues of the body. In the form of myoglobin, iron is found in all the muscles.

Functions of Iron:

1. As a part of respiratory pigment and heamoglobin, iron helps in the utilization of oxygen by the blood.

2. It activates enzymes by taking part in the enzyme system and assists in proper functioning of every organ of the body. Iron is also a component of many enzymes including cytochromes and certain flavoprotiens. 4 ppm iron is necessary for the formation of blood and growth of chicks.

Absorption and excretion: The amount of iron absorbed is related to its need by the animal body. The capacity of the body excrete the iron is very less therefore; its absorption is controlled by the body's requirement. There are two hypotheses for the control of iron absorption.

1. Mucosal Block theory: In this case iron is absorbed by the mucosal cells of gastro-intestinal tract, when they become physiologically saturated the iron absorption is checked.

2. The second mechanism by which iron absorption is controlled is the passage of iron from the mucosal cells to the stream which is controlled by the oxygen tension in the blood.

Before absorption, ferrous iron is oxidised to ferric state, following absorption into the mucosal cells there it binds with apoferritin, a protein, to form ferritin. At the blood stream end of mucosal cell the ferric iron is again converted into ferrous form and is detached from the ferrittin. In the blood stream it is again auto-oxidized and is attached to a protein siderophilin, in which form it is transported.

Factors which affect iron absorption:

1. Acidic condition in the gastro-intestinal tract helps iron absorption. Absorption of iron is more efficient when body stores are low.

2. Ascorbic acid in the diet also helps iron absorption.

3. High level of phosphorous and phytic acid present in the diet reduces iron absorption.

Deficiency symptoms: The deficiency symptoms of iron are lower weight gain, listleness, inability to withstand circulatory strain, laboured breathing after mild exercise, reduced appetite and decreased resistance to infection. Anaemia in piglets is characterized by poor appetite and growth. Breathing becomes laboured and spasmodic and this condition is called 'thump'.

Source of Iron: Milk is poor and green forages are rich sources of iron.

2. Copper: Copper is an integral part of cytochrome A and cytochrome oxidase. It appears that copper functions in the cytochrome system in the same way as iron, that is, through a change in valency. The enzymes tyrosinase, lactase, ascorbic acid oxidase, plasma amino oxidase, ceruloplasmin and uricase contain copper, and their activity is dependent on this element. Copper is present in blood plasma as a copper-protein complex, ceruloplasmin. Copper absorption takes place from the abomasums and small intestine. Dietary phytate, high levels of calcium carbonate, iron, zinc and molybdenum reduce absorption and excreted through faeces. Acidity of the stomach, intestinal secretion and the base content of the diet affect the absorption of copper from gasto-intestinal tract. In metabolism, copper is closely associated with molybdenum. Excess of molybdenum in the body result in poor absorption and storage of the copper salt. Deficiency of molybdenum causes more absorption and storage of the copper in the body.

Functions of copper:

1. Copper acts as catalyst in the formation of heamoglobin and provides oxygen absorption power to red blood cells.

2. As an essential part of enzymes system copper plays important role in various metabolic activities of the body.

3. The element is necessary for the normal pigmentation of hair, fur, wool and skin.

4. It is necessary for iron absorption from small intestine and iron absorption from tissue stores.

Deficiency symptoms: Copper deficiency includes anaemia, bone disorders , neonatal ataxia, depigmentation and abnormal growth of hair and wool, impaired growth and reproductive performance, retained placenta, heart failure, gastro intestinal disturbances, immunosuppression and lesions in the brain stems and spinal cord. These lesions are associated with muscular incoordination, and occur specially in young lambs.

Enzootic ataxia: The copper deficiency condition known as enzootic ataxia has been known for some time in Australia. The disorder is these associated with pasture low in copper content (2 to 4 mg/kg DM), and can be prevented by feeding with a copper salt.

Swayback: A similar condition which occurs in lambs occurs in U.K. called swayback. The symptoms of swayback in newborn lambs range from a complete inability to stand, to various degree of in-coordinationparticularly of the hind limbs.

Salt sick: For many years it had been recognized in Florida that cattle not thrive well due to copper deficiency. They lost their appetite. They become emaciated and weak and their blood was very low in heamoglobin. Young cattle were most affected and often badly stunted many of the animals died from the disease which is called salt sick.

Stringy wool (Steely wool, Falling disease, Baffing disease): Copper plays an important role in the production of crimp in wool. The element is present in an enzyme which is responsible for the disulphide bridge in two adjacent cysteine molecules. In the absence of enzyme the protein molecules of the wool donot form this bridge and referred as stringy or steely wool. This disease is called falling or baffing disease.

Falling disease: The disease is characterized by sudden death without any preliminary sign. In this fibrosis of myocardium takes place and macrocytic hypochromic type anaemia appears.

Coast disease (Neck ill, Lickin disease): This disease is caused by the deficiency of copper and cobalt in diet of cattle and sheep.

Teartness (Peat scours): Certain nutritional disease which are prevented or cured by copper supplement, the forage contains a normal amount of copper. However, the assimilation of copper is apparently prevented by an excess of another minerals. One disease is teartness, a type of sever scouring and unthriftiness which affects cattle pastured on certain area of England and similar conditions are noticed in New Zealand in peat soil pasture known as peat scour.

Sources of copper: The requirements of copper are quite difficult to determine since its absorption and utilization in the animal are markedly affected by several mineral elements and other dietary factors i.e. zinc, iron and molybdenum. Copper is widely distributed in feed. Some soils are deficient in copper in our country. Concentrates are rich sources of copper. Straws are poor source of copper. Cattle require 50 mg of copper per day. Moreover, requirement for sheep is 5 mg per day. Pigs require 5 ppm of copper per kg of diet per day.

Copper-Molybdenum-sulphur interrelation: Certain pasture on calcareous soils in part of England and Wales have been known to be associated with a condition in cattle described as 'teart' characterized by unthriftiness and scouring. A similar disorder occurs on reclaimed peat land in New Zealand, where it is known as peat scour. Molybdenum level in teart pasture are about 20 to 100 mg/kg DM compared to 0.5 to 3.0 mg/kg DM in normal pasture, and teart was originally regarded as being a molybdenosis. In the late 1930, however, it was demonstrated that feeding with copper sulphate controlled the scouring and hence a Molybdenum-copper relationship was established.

A mechanism which explains this interrelationship has recently been suggested. Sulphide is formed by ruminal microorganism from dietary sulphate or organic sulphur compounds; the sulphide then reacts with molybdate to form thiomolybdate which in turn combined with copper to form an insoluble copper thio-molybdate (Cu Mo Su) thereby limiting the absorption of dietary copper. In addition it is considered likely that if thiomolybdate is form in excess, it may be absorbed from the digestive tract and exert a systemic effect on copper metabolism in the animals.

3. **Iodine:** Iodine is found in thyroid gland where it is incorporated in the thyroxine, a hormone secreted by the gland. It is also a constituent of di-iodotyrosine.

Functions of Iodine:

1. Iodine is necessary for the proper functioning of the thyroid gland, treatment of simple goitre, control of metabolic activities and for the proper growth and development.

2. The thyroid hormone accelerates reactions in most organs and tissues in the body, thus increasing the basal metabolic rate, accelerating growth and increasing the oxygen consumption of the whole organism.

Absorption of iodine: Iodine is absorbed from the gastrointestinal tract. The rumen is the major site of absorption whereas abomasums is the major site of endogenous secretion or recently of circulatory iodine into the digestive tract. Iodine is excreted through urine.

Deficiency symptoms: The deficiency of iodine results in the development of simple goitre (enlargement of thyroid gland). In this condition the thyroxine production is reduced and so thyroid gland become over active and enlarged as a compensatory growth. The thyroid being situated in the neck, the deficiency condition in farm animals manifest itself as a swelling of the neck, 'big neck'.

In pigs, its deficiency causes falling of hair, rough and hard skin, reproductive failure, retarded growth rate, poor mental and sexual development.

Plants of Brassica family like cabbage, rape, kale and also soybeans, linseed, peas and groundnut are rich in goitrogens which cause the goitre even if the animals are receiving the adequate amounts of iodine intake.

Sources of iodine: Iodine is available in fish meal, cod liver oil and iodized salts such as sodium and potassium iodine.

4. Cobalt: Cobalt is dietary essencial for ruminants because it is necessary for the synthesis of vitamin B_{12} by the gastrointestinal microbes.

Functions of cobalt:

1. Cobalt is necessary for the growth and development of the body as well as for the multiplication of rumen microbes among ruminants.

2. It forms as essential part of the enzyme system and plays an important role in the synthesis of vitamin B_{12} in rumen. About 3 percent of ingested cobalt is converted into vitamin B_{12} in the rumen.

3. Cobalt is also involved in the synthesis of DNA and the metabolism of amino acids.

4. As a component of vitamin B_{12}, cobalt is involved in propionate metabolism where it acts as a cofactor.

Absorption of cobalt: Cobalt is utilized by rumen microbes in the rumen and also absorbed in the lower portion of the small intestine. Cobalt is mainly excreted in the faeces with small amount in urine.

Deficiency symptoms:

1. The deficiency of cobalt is seen among animals of that area (Australia and New Zealand) where pasture grass contain 0.04 to 0.07 ppm of cobalt. The ruminant animals suffer more as compared to other animals. Loss of appetite, emaciation, rough coat and paleness of skin, normocytic aneamià, retarted growth or weight loss, weakness and reproductive failure, stumping

gait and finally leading to death are the main symptoms of cobalt deficiency. In Australia and New Zealand, the deficiency of cobalt is called coast disease, enzootic marasmus, wasting disease, pining and vinguish etc.

In ruminants, cobalt is required by rumen microorganisms for the synthesis of vitamin B_{12}. Deficiency of cobalt leads to insufficient production of vitamin B_{12} to satisfy the animal requirements. These symptoms can be cured by the injection of vitamin B_{12} in the blood but the cobalt injection does improve the condition. Small amount of vitamin B_{12} also synthesized in caecum of monogatric animals but is not sufficient to meet the requirements of poultry and pigs.

Source of cobalt: Normally the feed and fodders contain traces of cobalt ranging from 0.1 to 0.25 ppm. Leguminous grasses are rich source of cobalt as compared to other animals feed. Cobalt sulphate and chloride are good source of cobalt. Cobalt has been reported to be toxic. Ingestion of 20-25 mg cobalt per 100 kg body weight daily may be toxic to the animals.

5. Zinc: Zinc has been found in very tissue in the animal body. It is found in higher concentration in skin, hair and wool than other tissue of the body. Zinc is a constituent of several enzyme systems in the body like carbonic dehydrogenase, pancreatic carboxypeptidase, glutamic dehydrogenase and a number of pyridine nucleotide dehydrogenases. In addition zinc act as a co-factors for many other enzymes.

Functions of Zinc:

1. Zinc is an important trace element for the proper growth of body and development of hairs and keratinization of epithelial tissues.

2. Being an essential part of insulin hormone it plays important role in the metabolism of carbohydrates. It is involved in the nucleic acid and vitamin A metabolism and protein synthesis.

3. Zinc play a key role in both cell and antibody mediated immune responses for resistant against infection and also provide protection against liver damage caused by toxins from the fungi.

Absorption of zinc: The zinc absorption takes place in small intestine. Absorption of zinc involves solubilisation of zinc, which is higher at high acidic pH, dissociation from the source, binding to receptors at the intestinal cell wall and transport into the cell aided by zinc binding proteins. The rate of absorption of zinc varies significantly between various forms within and between organic and inorganic sources (dietary level, amounts, chemical form of zinc). The inorganic sources have low solubility and poor dissociation and hence often pass through the gut into faeces without appreciable absorption. Zinc is mainly excreted through faeces and a small proportion through urine.

Deficiency symptoms:

1. **Zinc deficiency in cattle:** On the zinc deficient diet, milk production reduced, poor fertility, loss of hair, lower feed efficiency, loss of appetite etc.

2. **Zinc deficiency in calves:** Symptoms of zinc deficiency in calves include inflammation of the nose and mouth, stiffness of the joints, swollen feet and parakeratosis.

3. **Zinc deficiency in pigs:** Zinc deficiency in pigs is characterized by subnormal growth, depressed appetite, poor feed conversion efficiency and parakeratosis. The latter is a reddeing of the skin followed by eruption that develop in to scab. The deficiency symptoms are more common in young one and housed pigs fed ad libitum on a dry diet. High level of calcium in the diet aggravated the condition.

4. **Zinc deficiency in chicks:** Retarded growth, 'Frizzled' feather, parakeratosis and a bone abnormality referred to as the 'Swollen hock syndrome'.

Sources of Zinc: Brans are rich source of zinc. Feed and fodders contain adequate amount of zinc.

6. Manganese: The amount of manganese present in the animal body is very small, the highest concentrations occurring in the bones, liver, kidney, pancrease and pitutary gland. Excess amount of calcium and phosphorus in the body prevents its absorption from the digestive tract. The mineral is excreted out from the body along with bile in faeces and urine.

Functions of manganese:

1. Manganese plays an important role for the bone development and vital nutrient in the synthesis of chondroitin sulphate which is the organic matrix of the bone.

2. Manganese is important trace mineral for normal growth, reproduction, egg production and for the prevention of perosis among poultry.

3. Manganese is important in the animal body as enzyme activators such as phosphate transferases and decarboxylases associated with the Kreb's cycle.

4. This trace mineral has an active role in immune functions where it helps in detoxifying free oxygen radicals which can cause tissue damage produced by immune cells in response to killing bacteria.

Absorption of manganese: Manganese is one of the poorly absorbed and retained trace minerals in livestock. High dietary intake of calcium, phosphorous and iron reduces manganese absorption from the small intestine. The mineral is excreted out from the body along with bile in faeces and urine.

Deficiency symptoms:

1. **Cattle:** Deficiency of manganese show poor gowth, leg disorders, skeletal abnormalities, ataxia of the new born and reproductive failures.

2. **Swine:** In swine deficiency of manganese results in poor growth of bones with shortening of leg bones, enlarged hocks, muscular weakness, increase in back fat and irregular oestrus cycle.

3. **Poultry:** In young chicks a deficiency leading to perosis in young birds may be aggravated by high dietary intakes of calcium and phosphorus. Manganese deficiency in breeding birds reduces hatchability and causes retraction in chicks.

Sources of manganese: Forages are rich in manganese as

compared to cereals. In feed it is available in maize, oat, wheat, green fodder and brans.

7. Fluorine: The amount of fluorine in common feed stuffs is 1 to 2 part per million. Presence of 100 ppm fluorine in the ration on dry matter basis, and above 3 ppm in drinking water is toxic to animals.

Functions of Fluorine: In very small amount the mineral is essential for the growth and proper development of the bones and teeth. It reduces the incidence of dental caries.

Deficiency symptoms: Deficiency of fluorine causes dental caries.

Toxicity of fluorine: The major clinical signs of fluorine toxicity are found in teeth and bone. It is slowly being deposited in the body and produces ill effect afterward. The bone become thick and soft with dirty colouration, teeth loss their normal shining appearance. Finally they become soft and very weak. They look quite bad and are unable to bear cold water. Sometime yellow and black spots are also visible on the teeth. It results in loss of appetite, growth and production.

8. Selenium: The presence of selenium in roughages and concentrates is harmful to the animals. In soils it may be present upto 40 ppm. Selenium is present in all cells of the body but concentration is normally less than 1 ppm. Toxic concentration in liver and kidney are normally between 5 and 10 ppm. Most important role of selenium in livestock is prevention of liver necrosis in rat and exudative diathesis in chicks.

Functions of Selenium:

1. Selenium is essential for growth, reproduction, prevention of various diseases and protection of the integrity of tissues. The metabolic function of selenium is closely related with vitamin E and acts as an antioxident and required for adequate immune response.

2. It is essential for prostaglandin synthesis and essential fatty acid metabolism.

3. It has a strong tendency to complex with heavy metals and exerts a protective effect against the heavy metals.

4. Selenium is important part of an enzyme glutathione peroxidase. This enzyme destroys peroxides before they can damage body tissues.

5. Selenium is also important in sulphur amino acid synthesis. Sulphur amino acids protect animals against several diseases associated with low intakes of selenium and vitamin E. This protection is due to the antioxidant activity of selenium.

Deficiency symptoms:

1. Deficiency of selenium in the diet causes myopathies in sheep and cattle.

2. In hens selenium deficiency reduces hatchability and egg production. Exudative diathesis, a haemorrhagic disease of chick and dietary liver necrosis in pigs are prevented by either selenium or vitamin E.

3. Bilateral paleness and dystrophy of the skeletal muscle, mottling and dystrophy of myocardium (mulberry heart disease) are noticed in pigs. Mulberry heart disease is most common when cereal based diets contain less than 0.05 ppm selenium.

Toxic effect: Selenium toxicity is known as 'alkali disease' and 'blind staggers'. Which is characterized by stiffness of joints, lameness, loss of hair from mane and tail and skin lesions on the legs. In some parts of Haryana and Punjab, the animals suffer with selenosis, the disease is known as Degnala.

9. Molybdenum: This mineral is available in pasture grasses, liver, intestinal tissues and milk of the animals.

Functions of Molybdenum:

1. As a component of the enzyme xanthineoxidase, especially important to poultry for uric acid formation.

2. As a constituent of nitrate reductase it also helps in the utilization of nitrate.

3. It also takes parts in purine metabolism and stimulates action of rumen microorganism.

4. Molybdenum participates in the reaction of the enzyme with cytochrome C and also facilitates the reduction of cytochrome C by aldehyde oxidase.

Absorption of molybdenum: Molybdenum is absorbed from the intestine. It is excreted through urine with a small amount in bile and milk.

Deficiency symptoms: Deficiency symptoms under natural condition have not been reported.

Toxic effect: In the molybdenum toxicity (molybdenosis) in ruminants suffer from extreme diarrhoea, loss in weight and reduced milk yields. The condition is known as teartness.

10. Chromium: Chromium has been found in nucleoproteins isolated from beef liver and also in RNA preparation. It may play a role in the maintenance of the configuration of the RNA molecule. Chromium has also been shown to catalyze the phospho-glucomutase system activates the succinic dehydrogenase-cytochrome system. Chromium influences metabolism of glucose, lipid and protein. Chromium is a primary active component of glucose tolerance factor (GTF) which makes the metabolic action of hormone insulin, more effective in regulating energy utilization, muscle tissue deposition, fat metabolism and serum cholesterol levels. As an integral part of GTF, it helps in binding insulin to cell membrane receptors sites and subsequent transport of glucose and amino acids in side the cells.

Interaction of minerals: Minerals may interact with each other and with other nutrients and non-nutrient factors. This interaction is of two types:

1. Synergistic interaction: The interaction elements, which mutually enhance their absorption in the digestive tract and meet out the requirements of the body, are called synergistic interaction. The synergism of essential minerals is described as:

- Calcium is synergigm with phosphorous.
- Phosphorous with calcium, sulphur, iodine, copper and cobalt.
- Sodium, chlorine and potassium with each other.
- Sulphur with cobalt, magnesium and phosphorous.
- Zinc with molybdenum
- Manganese with copper, molybdenum, cobalt and iron.
- Copper with manganese, iodine, cobalt, iron and phosphorous.
- Iron with copper and manganese.
- Molybdenum with manganese and zinc.
- Magnesium with sulphur.
- Iodine with copper, cobalt and phosphorous.
- Cobalt with iodine, copper, manganese, sulphur and phosphorous.

Elements	Synergism with other minerals
Calcium	P
Phosphorous	Ca, S, Cu, I, Co
Sulphur	Co, Mg, P
Zinc	Mo
Manganese	Cu, Mo, Co, Fe
Copper	Mn, I, Co, Fe, P
Iodine	Cu, Co, P
Molybdenum	Mn, Zn
Cobalt	I, Cu, Mn, S, P
Iron	Cu, Mn
Magnesium	S

2. Antagonistic interaction: The interaction in which minerals inhibit the absorption of each other in the digestive tract and produce opposite effects on any biochemical functions is called antagonistic interaction. Antagonism may be one sided or two sided:

a. One sided antagonism: One-sided antagonism means one mineral is antagonize the other but other can not. Potassium inhibits the absorption of zinc and manganese but zinc and manganese may not.

Elements	Antagonism with other minerals
Calcium	Zn, Mn, Cu, I, Mg, Fe
Sodium	Zn, Mn
Chlorine	I
Sulphur	Cu, Se
Zinc	Co
Molybdenum	I, P
Potassium	Zn, P

b. Two sided antagonism: In two-sided antagonism both the mineral inhibit the function of each other. Phosphorous and zinc inhibit the absorption of each other. Similarly, zinc and copper antagonize with each other.

Elements	Antagonism with other minerals
Phosphorous	Zn, Mn, Fe, Mg
Zinc	Mo, Fe, P
Manganese	Mg, P
Copper	Zn, mo
Molybdenum	Cu, Zn
Iron	P
Magnesium	P, Mn

Interaction of minerals with other nutrients: Minerals are not only interacting with each other but also interact with other nutrients like protein, vitamins, carbohydrates, fats and feed additives like antibiotics, alkaloids, antioxidants and glucosides etc. Vitamin D affects the absorption of Ca, P, Mg and Zn. Vitamin E is anteracts with trace mineral selenium. The minerals may form new bonds with organic compounds and form chelates. Such mineral organic complex chelates may stimulate or inhibits the absorption of minerals.

- Fat affects the absorption of Mg and Ca.
- The protein level and their sources determine the degree of utilization of P, Mg, Zn, Cu and other minerals.

• Excess Mo stimulates the elimination of urea nitrogen and reduces the biosynthesis of muscle protein.

Specific deficiency of minerals:

Calcium: Ricket, Osteomalacia, Milk fever

Phosphorous: Ricket, Osteomalacia, Pica

Magnesium: Grass staggers, magnesium tetany

Iron: Anaemia, Thump

Copper: Enzootic ataxia, Sway back, Stringy wool

Iodine: Goiter

Cobalt: Coast disease, Wasting disease

Zinc: Parakeratosis in pig, Frizzled feather, Swollen hock syndrome

Manganese: Slipped tendon/ perosis (poultry)

Flourine: Dental caries

Selenium: Mulberry heart disease, Exudative diathesis, Tying up in horse

Toxicity:

Selenium: Alkali disease

Molybdenum: Teartness

Fluorine: Dental caries

Q.1. Fill in the blanks.

1. The Calcium deficiency symptoms are — — — — — — and — — — —.
2. Pica is deficiency symptoms of — — — — — — —.
3. Milk fever is deficiency symptom of — — — — — — —.
4. Gross staggers are deficiency symptoms of — — — — — — —.
5. Magnesium deficiency symptoms are — — — — C — — — — — — — —.
6. Deficiency symptoms of sodium are — — — and — — —.
7. The most commonly used source of sodium is — — — —.
8. The deficiency symptoms of chlorine are — — — — — and — — — — —.
9. Sulphur containing vitamins are — — — — — and — — —.
10. A hormone which contain sulphur is — — — — —.
11. Iron deficiency symptom is — — — — — — — —.
12. Enzootic ataxia is deficiency symptom of — — — — — —.

13. Stringy wool in sheep is deficiency symptom of — — — —.
14. Copper deficiency symptoms are — — — and — — — — —.
15. Goitre is deficiency symptoms of — — — — — — —.
16. Iodine deficiency results in — — — — — — —.
17. Cobalt is a component of vitamin — — — — —.
18. Swollen hock joint in chicks is deficiency symptoms of — — — —.
19. Manganese deficiency in poultry is — — — — — —.
20. Deficiency of fluorine is — — — — — — —.
21. Degnala disease is due to toxicity of — — — — — — — —.
22. Molybdenum toxicity in ruminants is known as — — —.
23. The selenium toxicity is also known as — — — — — — —.
24. Zinc shows one sided antagonism with— — — — — — — —.
25. Two minerals inhibits the absorption of each other is called— — — — — — — — — — —.
26. The interaction which mutually enhances their absorption in the digestive tract is called— — — — — — — — — — — — —.
27. Frizzled feather in chicks is due to deficiency of — — —.
28. "Big neck " is deficiency symptoms of— — — — — — — —.

Q.2. Explain the following:
1. General functions of minerals.
2. Mucosal block theory.
3. Deficiency symptoms of calcium and phosphorus.
4. Deficiency symptoms of magnesium and potassium.
5. Deficiency symptoms of sodium and chlorine.
6. Functions and deficiency symptoms of sulphur.
7. Functions of Iron.
8. Function and deficiency symptoms of copper.
9. Inter-relationship of copper-sulphur and molybdenum.
10. Deficiency symptoms of iodine and cobalt.
11. Deficiency sympotms of zinc, manganese and fluorine.
12. Deficiency symptoms of selenium, and molybdenum.
13. Inter-relationship of selenium and vitamin E.

Chapter 8

The Vitamins in Animal Nutrition

Definition of Vitamins:

Hofmeister defined vitamins as, these are substances, which are indispensable for the growth and maintenance of the animals, which occur both in animals and plants and are present in only small amounts in food.

In modern sense, vitamins are the substances distinct from major components of food required in minute quantities and whose absence causes specific deficiency disease. Plant can synthesize all the vitamins, which they require as a component of various enzyme systems. Vitamins are organic substances required by animals in very small amounts for regulating various body processes toward normal health, growth, production and reproduction. But this definition ignores the important part that these chemical substances found in plants and their importance generally in the metabolism of all living organisms.

The term vitamins was used by Funk in 1912 for an amine, the active factor from rice polishing which are necessary for existence of life (vital + amine). Later on the terminal "e" was omitted, leaving vitamin. The existence of vitamin like factors was first recognized in the orient when prisoners fed on unpolished rice seemed to be suffering with beri-beri disease than were non-prisoners consuming polished rice. Soon thereafter, workers in the United States recognized a factor in the butterfat of milk, which prevented blindness in calves. However, the factors seemed to be different from that in rice polishings since the milk fat factor was fat-soluble rather than water-soluble and also did not contain nitrogen.

There are atleast 15 vitamins, which has been accepted as essential food factors and few others have been proposed. The vitamins are divided into two main groups, the water-soluble and the fat-soluble, which are differentiated as:

	Parameters	Fat soluble vitamins	Water soluble vitamins
1.	Solubility	Fat soluble	Water soluble
2.	Chemical nature	Consist only of C,H, and O.	Ring compound except Pantothenic acid (straight chain), contains C,H,O,N,S,P or cobalt Vit. B_{12} contain cobalt, sulpher containing vitamins are thiamine and biotin
3.	Functions	Vit. A, D, E, K works as in vision, Calcium absorption, maintenance of genital system and blood clotting respectively	As coenzymes or prosthetic groups of enzymes except Vit. C.
4.	Synthesis	Only Vit. K is synthesized by symbiotic microorganisms Vit. D can be synthesized in the skin upon exposure to sun light	Ruminant synthesized all Vit. B complex with incorporation of cobalt in diet. Niacin can be synthesized from Tryptophane except cat. Vit. C except guinea pig. human.
5.	Absorption	Absorbed from gastro-intestinal tract by passive diffusion	Absorbed from gut directly
6.	Storage	Liver	Not stored except Vit. B_{12} (liver) and riboflavin (some extent)
7.	Excretion	Exertion in faeces via bile	Excreted in urine
8.	Toxicity	Excess dietary intake causes toxicity because they are stored in the body	Relatively non toxic

Functions of vitamins:

1.   Vitamins are essential for the good health and play important role in the body growth.

2. Vitamin provides resistance against diseases and increases the productivity power of animals.

3. Vitamins are essential constituents of certain enzyme systems, regulate body metabolism and clotting of blood.

4. Vitamins are needed during pregnancy for the development of foetus.

5. Vitamin 'A' is responsible for the proper functioning of vision and Vitamin C keeps the gums in healthy state.

Important vitamins in animal nutrition:

Vitamins	Chemical name
I. Fat soluble vitamins	
Vitamin A_1	Retinol
Vitamin A_2	Dehydroretinol
Vitamin D_2	Ergocalciferol
Vitamin D_3	Cholecalciferol
Vitamin E	Tocopherol
Vitamin K_1	Phylloquinone
Vitamin K_2	Menaquinone
Vitamin K_3	Menadione
II. Water soluble vitamins	
Vitamin B_1	Thiamin
Vitamin B_2	Riboflavin
Niacin	Nicotinamide
Vitamin B_6	Pyridoxine
Pantothenic acid	Pantothenic acid
Biotin	Biotine
Folacin	Folic acid
Choline	Choline
Vitamin B_{12}	Cyanocobalamin
Vitamin C	Ascorbic acid

Vitamin A: Vitamin A was discovered in 1913 by McCollum *et al.* It has been reported to occur in two different forms, *viz.* vitamin A_1 or retinol and vitamin A_2 or dehydroxyretinol. It is an unsaturated monohydric alcohol. One international unit of vitamin A is 0.344 μg of pure vitamin A acetate, which is equivalent to 0.3 μg of vitamin A alcohol. One

IU of provitamin A activity is equal in activity to 0.6 µg of β-carotene.

Chemical name: Vitamin A, known chemically as retinol, is an unsaturated monohydric alcohol with the following structural formula.

CH_3 CH_3

$$CH=CH-\overset{\overset{\displaystyle CH_3}{|}}{C}=CH-CH=CH-\overset{\overset{\displaystyle CH_3}{|}}{C}=CH-CH_2OH$$

CH_3

Vitamin A ($C_{20} H_{29} OH$)

Vitamin A does not exist as such in plants, but is present as precursors or pro-vitamin in the forms of certain carotenoid which can readily be converted into vitamin A by the animal. At least 80 provitamins are known and these included a,b and g carotenes, cryptoxanthine, which is present in higher plants and mycoxanthin which occur in the blue green algae. Provitamin β- carotene is the most widely distributed and most active. Vitamin A contains one b -ionone ring and b - carotene contains 2 β-ionone rings. Carotene is converted into vitamin A in the epithelial cell of intestine. Part of carotene is converted into vitamin A in the liver also.

Metabolism: Conversion of β-carotene to vitamin A takes place in intestinal mucosa. In most of animals absorption takes place in the form of vitamin A. Main site of vitamin A absorption is proximal jejunum. Liver is the main storage site of vitamin A (90 percent). In general, carotene digestibility was higher than average during warmer months and lower than average during winter.

Functions: Vitamin A plays following important functions.

1. **Growth:** Vitamin A is responsible for the normal development of various epithelial tissues in the body. Changes

have been demonstrated in the salivary gland, tongue and pharynx, respiratory tract, the genitourinary tract, eyes and certain glands of internal secretion. The primary change involves atrophy of the epithelium and the formation of stratified keratinizing epithelium.

2. **Vision:** Vitamin A is helpful in the transmission of light stumuli from the eye to the brain. Each vitamin A molecule is combined with specific type protein called opsin to form a visual pigment. Four such pigments have been identified which are rhodopsin and porpyropsin, which are present in rod and cyanopsin, which are in the cones of the retina. The rods are concerned with vision in dim light while the cones are concerned with bright light and colour vision.

3. **Reproduction:** Vitamin A plays an important role in male and female reproduction. Lack of vitamin A in the diet causes atrophy of the germinal epithelium resulting in sterlity.

4. **Skin:** Lack of vitamin A in the diet causing keratosis of the skin (dryness and roughness of skin). A keratosis especially of the hair follicles is a prominent feature.

5. **Urolithiasis:** A condition in which urinary calculi are present is known as urolithiasis. Lack of vitamin A in the diet causing keretinization of epithelial cells in genito-urinary tract followed by bacterial invasion and deposition of calcium phosphate precipitate on the site and ultimately calculi is formed.

6. **Infection:** Vitamin A has been called the anti-infective vitamin. The vitamin does help to establish and maintain a resistance to infection in the body, especially in tissues, which undergoes keratinization in a deficiency of it.

7. **Bone development:** Vitamin A has a role in the normal development of bone through a control activity of osteoclasts and osteoblasts of the epithelial cartilage.

Animal	Requirement (IU/Kg feed)
Beef cattle	2200-3800
Dairy cattle	2200-5000
Goat	5000
Chicken	1500-4000
Sheep	1500-2000
Swine	1400-2200
Horse	1600-2800
Dog	3300
Human children	400-700 µg/RE/day
Adults	800-1000µg/RE/day
Lactating	1200µg/RE/day

(Retinol equivalent (RE)= 1µg retinol or 6µg β-carotene)

Conversion of β-carotene to vitamin A

Animal	Conversion of mg of β-carotene to IU of vitamin A (mg) (IU)	IU of vitamin A activity (calculated from carotene) percent
Standard	1 = 1667	100
Beef cattle, Dairy cattle	1 = 400	24
Sheep		
Swine	1 = 500	30
Horse, Human	1 = 555	33.3
Poultry, Rat	1 = 1667	100
Cat, Mink	Carotene not utilized	

Factors influencing Vitamin A requirement: Follwing factors affect vitamin A requirements.

1. Genetic differences
2. Conversion efficiency of carotene to vitamin A
3. Variation in level, type and precursor of vit. A in feed stuff.
4. Destruction of vitamin A in feed through oxidation, peroxidizing effects of rancid fats, length of storage and catalytic effects of trace minerals.
5. Presence of adequate bile in small intestine.

Sources of Vitamin A: In the form of its precursor carotene, vitamin A is found in carrot, yellow maize and green plants. Liver, kidney, buttermilk, cod liver oil and egg yolk are also rich in vitamin A.

Vitamin A source	Vitamin A (IU/gram)
Whale liver oil	400,000
Cod-liver oil	4,000
Butter	35
Cheese	14
Eggs	10
Milk	1.5

Carotene source	Carotene (mg/Kg)
Alfalfa meal	110-300
Legume hay	10-60
Non Legume hay	20-30
Grains (except yellow corn)	0.20-0.44

Deficiency Symtpoms:

1. Night blindness: Diet deficient in Vitamin A causing impaired rhodopsin formation. Which make unable to see in dim light.

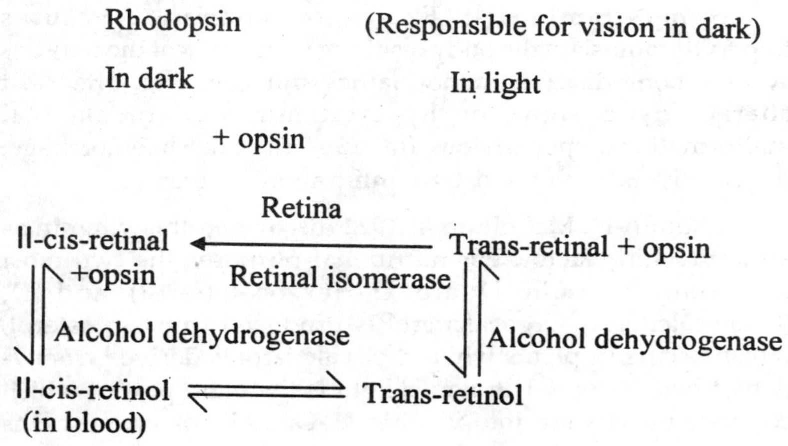

Rhodopsin   (Responsible for vision in dark)

In dark   In light

+ opsin

Retina

II-cis-retinal ⟵——————— Trans-retinal + opsin

  +opsin   Retinal isomerase

Alcohol dehydrogenase   Alcohol dehydrogenase

II-cis-retinol ⇌——⟶ Trans-retinol
(in blood)

Role of vitamin A in vision

137

2. Xerophthalmia: Cattle with prolonged eye symptoms leading to excessive watering, softening and cloudiness of the cornea and development of xerophthalmia, characterized by a drying of the conjunctiva. Constriction of the optic nerve canal may result in blindness in calves.

3. Infertility and abortion: In breeding animals a deficiency may lead to infertility, and in pregnant animals lead to abortion or the production of dead, weak and blind calves. In male there is failure of spermatogenesis.

4. Keratinization of epithelial cell: Vitamin A deficiency causes keratinization of epithelial cell, which results in cold and sinus trouble, diarrhea and formation of calculi in genito-urinary tract and reproductive failure in male and female animals.

5. Disorganized bone growth and irritation of joints are two manifestations of vitamin A deficiencies. In some cases, there is a constriction of the opening through which the optic and auditary nerves pass thereby resulting in blindness and / or deafness.

Poultry: Retarded growth, weakness, ruffled plumage and staggering gait are noticed in vitamin A deficiency. In mature birds egg production and hatchability are reduced.

Hypervitaminosis: Excess of vitamin A causes hypervitaminosis in the body resulting in diseases of the nervous system, bone diseases, abnormalties and vomiting. The most characteristic signs of hypervitaminosis are skeletal malformations, spontaneous fracture, interanal haemorrhage, degenrative atrophy and fatty infiltration of liver.

Vitamin-D: McCollum in 1922 discovered this vitamin as an antirachitic factor. For nutritional purposes the two most important vitamin D are D_2 (ergocalciferol) and D_3 (Cholecalciferol). Ergocalciferol is produced from ergosterol, which occurs in plants while cholecalciferol is derived from 7-dehydrocholesterol. Ultraviolet light is the main power, which converts provitamin into vitamin D. One I.U. of vitamin D is defined as the activity of 0.025µg crystalline vitamin D_3. The sulfate derivative of vit. D present in milk is a water-soluble form of vitamin. Vit. D_3 is more stable then D_2.

Metabolism:

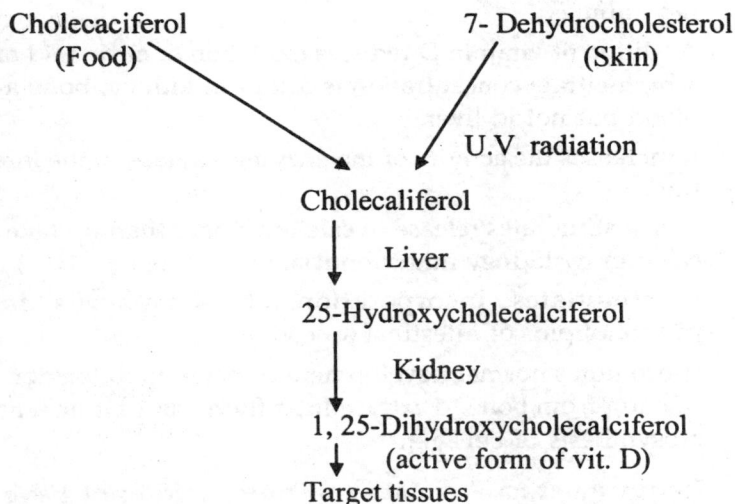

About 50 percent of the dietary vitamin is found in the chylomicrons leaving the digestive tract in the lymph; most of this vitamin finds its way to the liver with the remnants of the chylomicrons. Vitamin D synthesized in the liver diffuses into the blood and picked up by a specific vitamin D bind protein which transports it to the liver, although some may remain free and be deposited in fat and muscle. Dietary vitamins D_2 and D_3 are absorbed through the small intestine and are transported in the blood to the liver where they are converted into 25-hydroxycholecalciferol, which is converted into active form as 1, 25- dihydroxycholecalciferol in kidney and reached to target tissues by blood circulation. Vitamin D transported by protein called transcalciferin or vitamin D binding protein (DBP). Excretion of absorbed vitamin D and its metabolites occurs primarily in faeces with the addition of bile salts.

Functions:

1. Vitamin D plays an important role for the absorption of calcium and phosphorus from gastrointestinal tract, which accounts for the antirachitic properties of vitamin D.

2. It helps in the reabsorption of phosphorus from the kidney tubules.

3. Addition of vitamin D reduces oxidation of citric acid and a high citrate concentration is found in kidney, bone and blood but not in liver.

4. It increases the activity of the enzyme phytase in the intestine.

5. It also stimulates release of calcium rather than up take of calcium by kidney mitochondria.

6. It stimulates incorporation of phosphorus into phospholipids of intestinal mucosa.

7. It promotes normal development of bone, mobilization of calcium from bone to extracellular fluid compartment and biosynthesis of collagen.

Requirements: Animals and humans do not have a nutritional requirement for vitamin-D. Factors, which influence dietary vitamin D requirements are:

(i) Amount and ratio of dietary calcium and phosphorus.

(ii) Availability of phosphorus and calcium

(iii) Species

(iv) Physiological factors.

Animal	Requirement (IU/Kg feed)
Beef cattle	275
Dairy cattle	300
Goat	1400
Chicken	400
Swine	220
Dog	22 IU/Kg body weight
Sheep	550 IU/ 100kg live weight
Human	200-600 IU/day

Sources of vitamin D: As vitamin D it is present in cod-liver oil, kidneys, lungs, egg yolk, liver, milk, fish oil and sun dried grasses. The vitamin is synthesized by the action of ultra-violet rays on the skin of the animals. Heating destroys the rachitogenic activity.

Ergocalciferol (D₂)

Food or Feed stuff	IU/100gram
Alfalfa hay, sun cured	142
Barley straw	60
Corn silage	13
Molasses (sugar beat)	58
Red cloever, sun cured	192
Sorghum silage	66

Cholecalciferol (D₃)

Blue fin tuna liver oil	4,000,000
Cod liver oil meal	4,000
Cod liver oil	10,000
Halibut liver oil	1,20,000
Milk, cow whole	1-4

Deficiency Symptoms: Deficiency of vitamin D impairs the following functions.

(a) Failure of calcium salt deposition in the cartilage matrix.

(b) Failure of cartilage cells to mature, leading to their accumulation rather than destruction.

(c) Condensation of proliferating cartilage cells.

(d) Elongation, swelling and degeneration of proliferative cartilage.

(e) Abnormal pattern of invasion of cartilage by capillaries.

In young animal vitamin D deficiency results in rickets and retarded growth. Ricket includes skeletal deformities characterized by enlarged junction between bone and cartilages, curvature of the bones, tendency to drag hind legs, beaded ribs, deformed thorax and weakening of muscular tissue and susceptibility to infection. In adult animals vitamin D deficiency causes osteomalacia, where there is reabsorption of bone calcium already laid down.

In poultry a deficiency of vitamin D causes the bone and beak to become soft and rubbery, growth is usually retarded and the legs may become bowed, ruffled feathers. Egg production is reduced and egg quality deteriorates.

In swine, deficiency of vitamin D causes poor growth, stiffness, lameness and stilted gait, softness of bones, bone deformities, unthriftiness, enlargement and erosion of joints.

Hypervitaminosis of vit D₃:

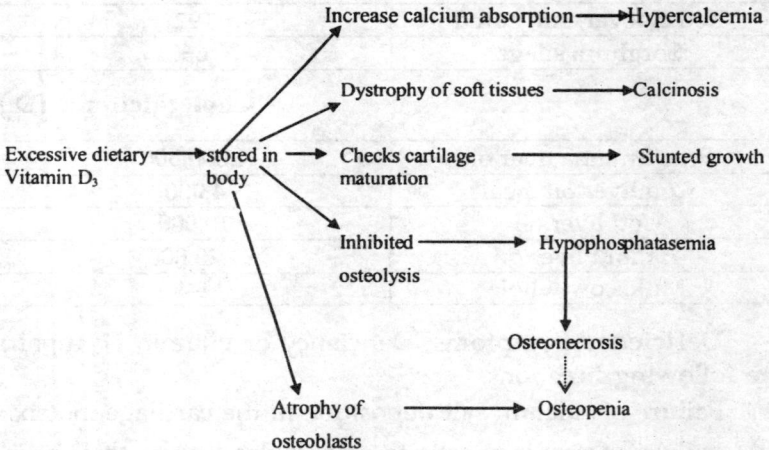

Vitamin-E (Tocopherol): In 1936 Evans and Sure discovered it as an important factor in reproduction of rats. After absorption from the wall of the gastrointestinal tract the vitamin is mainly stored in the liver and to a certain extent in various organs and tissues of the body. The vitamin can pass through the placenta and mother's milk to its offsprings. Vitamin E is a group name, which includes a number of closely related active compounds. Eight naturally occurring forms of the vitamins are known and they can be divided into two groups.

1. Four saturated vitamins that is a, b, g and d tocopherols
2. Four unsaturated vitamins that is a, b, g and d tocotrienols,

α-tocopherol is the most biologically active and most widely distributed. Selenium and vitamin E are interrelated. Both are needed by animals and both have metabolic roles in the body in addition to an antioxidant effect.

Metabolism: It acts as a biological antioxidant with glutathione peroxidase enzyme, which contains selenium. It protects cells against oxidative damage caused by free radicals. Free radicals are scavenged by vitamin E and glutathione peroxidase destroys any peroxide formed before they can damage the cell. Vitamin E is also helpful in development and function of the immune system. Absorption of Vit.E either in free alcohol or esters is facilitated by bile and pancreatic lipase. Most of Vit.E is absorbed as alcohol. Tocopherol passes through placental membranes and mammary gland. Less than 2 percent of dietary Vit.E is transferred from feed to milk. Vit. E is stored through out all body tissues, with highest storage in liver. In the plasma, the vitamin is transported in the low density lipoprotein (LDL) fraction and concentrates in the cell membrane. Highest concentrations are found in the adipose tissue, other organs and tissues which contain the vitamin include liver, heart, skeletal muscle and adrenal gland.

Functions:
1. Vitamin E acts as an antioxidant at cellular level. Thus for an example it prevent the oxidation of unsaturated fatty acids mostly present in all cell wall components. a-tocopherol is an excellent natural antioxidant.

2. It participates in normal tissue respiration possible by the way of cytochrome reductase system and to protect the lipid structure of mitochondria from oxidative destruction.

3. It aids the normal phosphorylation of creatine phosphate, ATP-which is a high phosphate energy compound in the body.

4. It also involved in the synthesis of ascorbic acid, ubiquinone (Co-enzyme) and the metabolism of nucleic acid.

5. α-tocopherol exerting a unique influence on structural component of membrane phospholipid.

6. It stimulates the formation of prostoglandin E from arachidonic acid while synthetic vit. E had no effect.

7. Vit. E inhibits platelet aggregation so help in blood clotting.

8. Relationship of vit E with toxic elements-

Both vitamin E and selenium provide protection against toxicity with three groups of heavy metals.

(i)   Cadmium and Mercury- Selenium is highly effective in altering toxicities, vit. E has little influence.

(ii) Silver and Arsenic- Vit. E is highly effective and selenium at higher doses.

(iii) Lead- Vit. E is highly effective in altering toxicity produced by lead.

Requirements: Vit. E requirement of normal animals and humans is approximately 30 ppm of diet. Requirement of vit E is dependent on dietary levels of polyunsaturated fatty acids (PUFA), antioxidants, and sulphur containing amino acids and selenium.

Animal	Requirement (IU/Kg animal feed)
Beef cattle	15-60
Dairy cattle	300
Goat	100
Chicken	5-10
Turkey	10-25
Sheep	15-20
Swine	10-20
Dog	22
Horse	233 µg/Kg body weight
Human	8-13 mg/day

Sources: Vitamin E is widely distributed in foods. Green fodder is good sources of α-tocopherol. Cereal grains are also good sources. Animal products are relatively poor sources of the vitamin. One I.U. of vitamin E is defined as the specific activity of 1mg synthetic α-tocopherol acetate.

Feed and Feed stuff	α-tocopherol content of feed (ppm)
Alfalfa meal, dehydrated 17% protein	30-120
Alfalfa meal, sun cured, 13% protein	18-60
Alfalfa hay	23-102
Barley, whole	22-42
Butter	10-33
Egg	8-12
Oat	18-24
Rice bran	34-87
Wheat bran	15-20
Sorghum grain	10-16

Deficiency symptoms: The vit E deficiency symptoms in farm animals are muscle degeneration (myopathy). Nutritional myopathy (muscular dystrophy) in cattle affects the skeletal muscles, which is manifested by difficulty in standing, trembling and staggering gait. The animals are unable to rise and weakness of the neck muscles prevents them from raising their heads, also known as white muscle disease. Nutritional myopathy in lambs is called stiff lamb disease (white muscle disease).

In pigs vitamin E deficiency diseases are myopathy and cardiac disease known as mulberry heart disease (haemorrhagic lesions within the heart that gives characteristic 'mulberry' appearance) and hepatosis dietetica (toxic liver dystrophy). In poultry, Vit. E defciency causes following diseases.

1. **Exudative diathesis:** It is characterised by edema, blackening of affected part, apathy and inappetance.

2. **Nutritional encephalomalacia (Crazy chick disease):** It is characterised by ataxia, head retraction and cycling with legs.

3. Muscular dystrophy

* Vitamin E is non toxic even at higher doses.

Vitamin-K: Vitamin-K was identified in 1935 by Henrik Dam to be an essential factor in the prevention of haemorrhagic symptoms produced in chicks. The new fat-soluble vitamin was designated as vitamin K for the Danish word Koagulation. Vitamin K is synthesized in the body of ruminants by the action of rumen microbes. Bile juice assists in the absorption of this vitamin from the intestine. In dogs there is microbial synthesis in the intestine. The important naturally occurring compounds are vitamin K_1 (Phylloquinone) and vitamin K_2 (Prenyl-menaquinone). Vitamin K_3 (Menadione) is a synthetic compound, which is about 3.3 times as potent, biologically, as the naturally occurring vitamin K_2.

Metabolism: Like all fat-soluble vitamins, Vitamin K is absorbed in association with dietary fats and requires the presence of bile salts and pancreatic juice for adequate uptake from the alimentary canal vit. K is stored in the liver. Most of the ingested vitamin appears in the chylomicrons entering the lymph. The synthetic form is absorbed directly in the hepatic portal vein and carried to the liver, where it is activated and then released along with the naturally occuring forms of vitamin K. These are carried in the LDL to target sites.

Functions: The vitamin K is necessary for the formation of prothormbin, which is important intermediate of the blood clotting process. Prothrombin must bind to calcium ions before it can be activated as thrombin. If the supply of vitamin K is inadequate, the prothrombin molecule is deficient in a-carboxyglutamic acid, a specific amino acid responsible for calcium binding. Thrombin converts the protein fibrinogen in blood plasma into fibrin, which holds blood clots together. There are four blood clotting proteins, which are dependent on vitamin K for their synthesis.

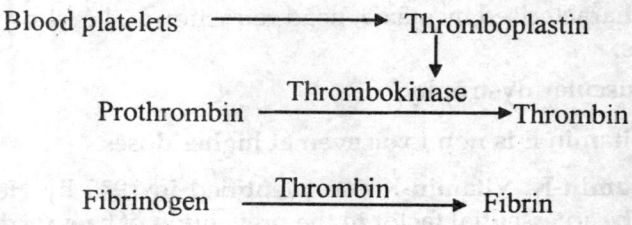

146

The important biochemical function has been found to be involved in electron transport and in bacteria, oxidative phosphorelation.

Requirements: The daily requirement for most species varies in a range of 2-200 μg vitamin K /Kg body weight. This requirement can be altered by age, sex, strain, antivitamin K factor, disease condition.

Animal	Requirement (mg/Kg)
Beef cattle, Dairy cattle, Horse, Goat, Sheep	Microbial synthesis
Swine	0.5
Fish	0.5-1.0
Dog	1.0
Chicken	0.5-1.0
Human Infants Adult	 12μg/day 70-140 μg/day

Sources of Vitamin K: Green and leafy fodder, Lucerne, Cabbage, soyabean, liver, fish meal and egg yolks are good source of vitamin K.

Feed or feed stuff	Vit K level (ppm)
Alfalfa hay, sun cured	19.4
Alfalfa dehydrated	14.2
Spinach	6.0
Tomato	4.0
Barley, corn, sorghum, grains	0.2
Liver	1-8
Milk (cattle)	0.02
Milk (human), Egg	0.2
Fish meal	2.2

Deficiency symptoms:

1. Ruminants and pigs: Under normal conditions vitamin K deficiency have not been reported, but deficiency symptoms, occur when spoiled sweet clover forage is fed. When sweet clover hay undergoes spoilage with certain molds, the coumarin is converted to dicumarol, (Dicumarol passes through the placenta in pregnant animals and new born animals may become affected immediately after birth) an anti-vitamin K and lowers the prothrombin content of the blood and at the same time a bleeding syndrome develops throughout the animal body. This disease is called sweet clover poisoning or bleeding diseases or haemorrhagic sweet clover disease. Prolongation the prothrombin time in absence of liver disease indicates vitamin K deficiency. Initial signs may be stiffness and lameness from bleeding into the muscles and articulations. Haematomas, epistaxis or gastrointestinal bleeding may be observed.

2. Poultry: The symptom of vitamin K deficiency in chicks is a delayed clotting time of the blood; birds are easily injured and may bleed to death. Chicks show anaemia, which in part may be due to loss of blood or to the development of a hypoplastic bone marrow.

3. Human: It is uncommon in humans because wide distribution of vitamin K in plant and animal tissue and microflora of gut synthesize the menaquinones. Newborn infants may suffer because-

(i)   Placenta is a relatively poor organ for maternal-foetal transmission of lipids.

(ii)   Sterile gastrointestinal tract.

(iii) Breast and cow's milk are poor source of vitamin K.

Factors which causes vit. K deficiency:

1.   Increase control feeding with less pasture and alfalfa meal.

2.   Feeding of solvent extrcted soyabean meal and other seed meal and better quality fishmeal.

3.   Haemorragic gastric ulcers which occurs frequently.

4.   Mycotoxins and molds present in the feed.

5. Any antimetabolites (antivitamin K) in the feed.
6. Use of sulfa drugs and different type of antibiotics.
7. Use of slatted floors which reduce the opportunity for coprophagy.

Vitamin K toxicity: Toxic effects mainly related with haematological and circulatory disturbances. The natural vitamin K phylloquinone and menaquinone are non-toxic at very high dose level. Synthetic menadione shows toxic effects at higher level i.e. anaemia, hemoglobinuria and urobilinuria.

Water soluble vitamins: The vitamins of the B complex and vitamin C comprise the water soluble group. Vitamin C is the only member of the water soluble groups that is not a member of the B family and its functions and characteristics are different from the B complex vitamins.

Vitamin B Complex: The vitamins included under this group are water soluble and most of them a component of co-enzymes. Ruminants are able to synthesis all the vitamin of B group in the rumen through rumen microorganism. In pre-ruminant calves and mono gastric animals B-complex vitamin should be supplied in the daily ration.

Some coenzymes and enzyme prosthetic groups involving the B vitamins:

Vitamin	Co-enzyme or prosthetic group	Enzymatic and other function
Thiamine	Thiamin diphosphate (TDP), Thiamin pyrophosphate	Oxidative decarboxylation
Riboflavin	Flavin mononucleotide (FMN), Flavin adenine dinucleotide (FAD)	Hydrogen carrier
Nicotinamide	Nicotinamide adenine dinucleotide and their phosphate	Hydrogen carrier
Pyridoxine	Nicotinamide adenine dinucleotide phosphate (NADP)	Transaminases and decarboxylases
Pantothenic acid	Co-enzyme (Co A)	Acyl transfer
Folic acid	Tetrahydrofolic acid	One carbon transfer
Biotin	Biotin	Carbondioxide transfer
Cyanocobalmin	Methyl cobalmin	Isomerases and dehydrases

Thiamin (Vitamin B₁): Thiamin is considered to be the oldest vitamin. Deficiency of this causes beri-beri in man which is earliest documented deficiency disorder. In 1890 Eiijkman, a Dutch investigator, seen polynerritis in chicken that was fed boiled polish rice. Jansen and Donath (1926) succeeded in crystallizing vitamin B in pure form. In 1936 R.R. Williams determined the chemical structure of thiamin. I.U. of thiamin is the activity of 3 µg thiamine hydrochloride. Thiamin is a complex nitrogenous base containing a pyrimidine ring joined to a thiazole ring. Because of the presence of hydroxyl group at the end of the side chain, thiamine can form esters. The main form of thiamine diphosphate ester (TDP) formerly known as thiamine pyrophosphate (TPP), although thiamine monophosphate and thiamine triphosphate are also occure.

Metabolism: Thiamine is absorbed in duodenum. Ruminants can also absorb free thiamin from the rumen. The horse can also absorb from the caecum. The mechanism of thiamin absorption is both active absorption and simple diffusion. At high levels of intake, most absorption is passive. Absorption may be inhibited by alcohol and by the presence of thiaminases, which are found in some fishes. On absorption, thiamine is phosphorylated to thiamine pyrophosphate (TPP), especially in the liver. The major tissues which contain thiamine are the skeletal muscle, heart, liver, kidney and brain. Thiamin is most poorly stored of all vitamins, is mainly retained in organs with a high metabolic activity. Absorbed thiamine is mainly excreted through urine, faeces and sweat.

Functions: Thiamine diphosphate is a coenzyme involved in the oxidative decarboxylation of pyruvic acid to acetyl coenzyme A, the oxidative decarboxylation of á–ketogluterate to succinyl coenzyme A in TCA cycle the pentose phosphate pathway. Thiamine involved in the synthesis of the amino acid valine in bacteria, yeast and plants.

Deficiency symptoms: Deficiency of thiamin in human causes beri-beri disease, which is characterised by numbness of the legs, later with pain in muscles, severe exhuastion, finally emaciation and paralysis. The patients have difficulty in breathing, there is an abnormal enlargement of the right side of the heart and decrease in the rate of the heart beat. The most characteristics feature of the disease is the so-called pheripheral neuritis. This is often accompanied by contraction of the feet and severe weakness of the wrists. The brain may be affected under these conditions.

Thiamine deficiency in chick causes poor appetites and consequently emaciated followed by polyneuritis, which is characterised by nerve degeneration paralysis. On thiamin deficient animals, there is an accumulation of pyruvic acid and its reduction product, lactic acid, in their tissues, which leads to muscular weakness. Ruminants since microbial synthesis occur in the rumen of cattle, sheep and goat and in the caecum of horses are unlikely to show thiamin deficiency. Raw fish contains thiaminase, which destroys the activity of thiamin of food with which the raw fish is mixed. Heat treatment or cooking destroyed the activity of thiaminase. Microbes of gastro-intestinal tract of man, pig, poultry, cat and dogs are having thiaminase activity. Due to this reason the thiaminase deficiency occurs.

Sources: Egg yolk, liver, heart, all living cells of the body, milk, meat, green grasses, cereal grains and yeast are rich sources of this vitamin.

Riboflavin (Vitamin B$_2$): It was found in a coenzyme before it was discovered in free form. The discovery of riboflavin goes back to 1929 when Norris and his associates found out an unknown vitamin as a cause of leg paralysis among chicks. In 1934 Gyorgy isolated it from B complex. Independently, Kuhn and Karrer *et al.* (1935) synthesized it. Riboflavin consists of a dimethyl-isoalloxazine nucleus combined with ribitol. It is yellow, crystalline compound and soluble in water. It is stable in heat, acid and nerutal solution but destroyed by alkali. It is unstable to ultraviolet light.

Absorption and metabolism of Riboflavin: Riboflavin is readily absorbed from the small intestine. In the plasma it is carried in association with albumin, which carries both the free vitamin and co-enzyme forms. In the tissues, riboflavin is converted into co-enzymes flavin mononucleotide (FMN) and flavin adenine dinucleotide, which constitute the active groups in a number of flavoproteins.

Functions: Riboflavin is required as part of many enzymes essential to utilization of carbohydrate, protein and fats. Riboflavin in the form of flavin mononucleotides (FMN) and Flavin adenine dinucleotide (FAD) act as the prosthetic group of several enzymes involves in biological oxidation-reduction reaction. Both FMN and FAD act as electron and hydrogen donors and acceptors, which allow them to play a critical role in many oxidation-reduction reactions of metabolic pathways, passing electron to the electron transport chain.

Deficiency symptoms: Deficiency of riboflavin in human produces a cheilosis (severe dermatitis and fissures at the corner of the mouth), angular stomatitis, glossitis and seborrheic dermatitis.

Chick: Deficiency causes slow growth and develops "curled toe paralysis" a specific symptom, caused by peripheral nerve degeneration, in which the chicks walk on their hocks with toe curled inwards. In breeding hen causes poor hatchability, embryonic abnormalities, including characteristic "clubbed down" condition in which the down feathers continue to grow inside the follicle, resulting in a coiled feather.

Sources: It is widely distributed throughout the plant and animal kingdom with very rich sources in anaerobic fermenting bacteria. Milk, liver, kidney and heart are good sources of vitamin.

Niacin (Nicotinamide): American scientist Elvehjem and his associates in 1937 discovered this vitamin as a cure for black tongue disease in dogs and pellagra in human being. It is not destroyed by heat, acid, alkali or by oxidation.

Absorption and metabolism of niacin: There is a rapid absorption of dietary niacin, both by active and passive mechanisms. Once the niacin has been converted to NAD or NADP, it is trapped within the cells and can not diffuse out.

NAD and NADP act as hydrogen acceptors in oxidation reactions forming NADH and NADPH.

Functions: Its function in the animal body as coenzyme such as: Diphosphophyridine nucleotiede (DPN) or coenzyme I or Nicotinamide adenine dinucleotide (NAD) and Triphosphophyridinenucleotide (TPN) or coenzyme II or NADP (Nicotinamide adenine dinucleotide phosphate (NADP).

The primay action of these two coenzymes is to remove hydrogen from substrate as a part of dehydrogenase enzymes and transfer hydrogen and/or electrons to the next coenzyme in the chain or to another substrate which then become reduced.

Deficiency symptoms:

Poultry: The deficiency of vitamin causes "black tongue" characterized by inflammation of the mouth and the upper part of the oesophagus. In chick deficiency produces enlargement of the tibiotarsal joint, a bowing of the legs, poor feathering and slight dermatitis.

Swine: In swine niacin deficiency is known as "pig pellagra" the disease is characterized by poor growth, poor hair and skin condition, occasional vomiting and diarrhoea.

Sources: Nicotinic acid can be synthesized from tryptophan in the body tissues. Niacin is found abundantly in yeast, meat, liver and poultry, groundnut and sunflower meal, milk, tomatoes and varieties of leafy green vegetables. Milk and eggs are almost deviod of the vitamin alothough they contain the precursor tryptophan.

Pyridoxine (Vitamin-B$_6$): Pyridoxine was first defined by Gyorgy (1934) as a part of vitamin B-complex, which is responsible for specific dermatitis in rats. The dermatitis is characterized by scaliness around the peripheral part of the body such as paws and mouth. The vitamin exists in three forms (pyridoxine, pyridoxal and pyridoxamine) which are interconvertible in the body tissues. The amine and aldehyde derivatives are less stable than pyridoxine and are destroyed by heat.

Absorption and metabolism of vitamin B$_6$: The vitamin has to be released from its phosphorylated forms prior to absorption. Once in its free form, absorption is rapid. The liver and muscles are the main sites for pyridoxal phosphate in the body; once it is phosphorylated, the vitamin is trapped in the cell. Pyridoxal is involved in many biological reactions particularly those associated with amino acid metabolism like decarboxylation and transamination etc.

Functions: The active compound pyridoxal phosphate plays an essential role as a coenzyme in the reaction by which a cell transforms nutrient amino acids into mixture of amino acids and other nitrogenous compounds required for its own metabolism. These reactions involve the activities of transaminases and decarboxylases.

Requirement:

Animals	Requirements
Ruminants and horse	Microbial synthesis
Chicken	3.0-4.5 mg/kg
Rat	6.0 mg/kg
human	0.3-2.8 mg/kg

Sources: Yeast, liver, milk, pulses and cereal grains are rich sources of this vitamin. To a limited extent egg and leafy vegetables are also a source of vitamin.

Food and food stuffs	Vitamin B$_6$ (mg/kg)
Alfalfa sun cured	4.4
Lin seed meal	6.0
Barley grain	7.3
Wheat bran	9.6
Corn	5.3-8.8

Deficiency symptoms:

Chicks: IPyridoxine deficiency causes acute convulsion, flatter on the pen, usually start kicking, a characteristic pasture with wings slightly spread and head resting on ground and generally die.

Pigs: Deficiency of vitamin causes anorexia, roughness of hair coat, fatty infiltration of the liver, goose step type of gait and convulsions:

Pantothenic Acid: Williams and his associates discovered pantothenic acid in 1933 which was derived from Greek word "pantos" means found every where. Pantothenic acid is a dipeptide derivative and the two components of pantothenic acid are dihydroxydimethyl-butyric acid and the amino acid, β-alanine.

Functions: Pantothenic acid is the prosthetic group of coenzyme A, an important coenzyme involved in many reversible acetylation reactions in carbohydrate, amino acid and fat metabolism with synthesis of steroids. Coenzyme A may act as an acetyl donor and acetyl acceptor. The vitamin involved in the formation of citrate oxaloacetate in the T.C.A. cycle.

Requirement: For growth and reproduction, the majority of species have a dietary requirement between 5 and 15 mg/kg. For egg production by chickens the vitamin requirement is very low (2.2 mg/kg) compared to requirement of 10 mg/kg for growth and reproduction.

Animals	Requirement
Ruminants and horse	Microbial synthesis
Swine	12 mg/kg
Human	4-7 mg/kg

Sources: Egg yolk, kidney, liver and yeast, groundnuts, pea skimmed milk, sweet potatoes and molasses are the good source of this vitamin.

Food and food stuffs	Pantothenic acid (mg/kg)
Alfalfa hay, sun cured hay	28-32
Mollases, sugar cane	50
Barley grain	9
Brewer's grain	9
Butter milk cattle	40
Eggs	27
Fish meal	1
Liver	165

Deficiency symptoms: It causes severe degeneration of myelin sheath of nervous tissues and affects steroid hormones of adrenal gland.

Poultry: Retarded growth, dermatitis, fatty liver condition, severe edema and subcutaneous haemorrhage are the common symptoms.

Swine: Deficiency symptoms are retarted growth rate and bloody diarrhea. Goose stepping gait, a typical nerve disease that is characterized by movement of hind leg become stiff and jerky, exaggerated legs.

Folic Acid (Folacin): The name folic acid was proposed by Mitchell *et al.* (1941) for a compound isolated from spinach and shown to be necessary for growth of streptococcus faecelis R. The same pterayl glutamic acid compound was later on called as folic acid. It contains three distinct components i.e. p-amino benzoic acid (PABA) and pteridine nucleus.

Absorption and metabolism of folate: Most folate in the diet is in the bound form and for optimal absorption glutamates have to be removed to produce the monoglutamate. Most folate is stored in the liver, which is therefore also a good dietary source of folate. Once taken up by target cells, polyglutamates are formed. These are trapped within the cell and are used as co-enzyme tetrahydroforate. Polyglutamate forms are digested via hydrolysis to pteroyl monoglutamate prior to transport across the intestinal mucosa. The enzyme responsible for the hydrolysis of pteroyl polyglutamate is a "ā-carboxy peptidase" known as folate conjugate. Pteroyl polyglutamate is absorbed predominately in the duodenum and jejunum by an active process involving sodium.

Functions: The active form of the vitamin is tetrahydrofolic acid (FH_4), Folic acid is carrier for the single carbon groups, may be either formyl (-CHO), formate (H. COOH), or hydroxymethyl ($-CH_2OH$). These are metabolically interconvertible in a reaction catalyzed by a NADP dependent hydroxymethyl dehydrogenase. Folic acids are important in the biosynthesis of purine and pyrimidines and in certain methylation reactions. Folic acid is involved in the interconversion of glycine to serine, methylation of ethanolamine to choline and homocysteine to methionine. Folic acid is needed to maintain immune system.

Requirement:

Animal	Requirement (mg/kg)
Ruminants	Microbial synthesis
Chicken	0.25-0.50
Swine	0.30
Dog	0.20
Horse	20 mg/day
Human	40-800 µg/day

Sources: Fresh leafy green vegetables, cauliflower, cereals and extracted oilseeds meal are rich sources of folic acid.

Feed and feed stuffs	Folacin (mg/kg)
Alfalfa meal	5.5
Brewer's grain	7.7
Cabbage, corn	0.3
Fish meal	0.2
Liver	8.4
Rice polish	0.2
Linseed meal	1.4

Deficiency symptoms: Glossitis, gastrointestinal disturbances, diarrhoea and reduced erythropoiesis are common deficiency symptoms. In chicks, poor growth, poor feathering, depigmentation, anaemic appearance and perosis develops. In pigs, macrocytic anaemia, lipopenia, megaloblastic arrest etc. develops.

Biotin: Biotin was first described as the factor protective against "egg white injury". Egg white contains avidine which combined with biotin and prevent its absorption from the intestine. Chemically, biotin is 2-keto-3, 4-imidazolido-2-tetrahydro-thiophene-n-valeric acid. Rat fed large amount of raw egg white devloped an eczema-like dermatitis, paralysis of the hind legs, and characteristics alopecia around the eyes, aptly termed spectacle eye. This vitamin has been known by a variety of names including bios factor, vitamin-H, coenzyme R and egg white injury protection factor.

Functions: Biotin serves as the prosthetic group of several enzymes which catalyze fixation of carbon dioxide into organic linkage. Enzymes containing biotin include acetyl coenzyme A carboxylase, propionyl coenzyme A carboxylase and methylmalonyl transcarboxylase. The acetyl coenzyme A carboxylase is required for the initial stage of fatty acid synthesis. In biological systems, it function as the coenzyme for carboxylases, enzyme which catalyse carbon dioxide fixation or carboxylation and also appear to be necessary for synthesis of dicarboxylic acids. Specific biotin dependent reactions in carbohydrate metabolism are-

1. Carboxylation of pyruvic acid to oxaloacetic acid
2. Conversion of malic acid to pyruvic acid
3. Interconversion of succinic acid and propionic acid
4. Conversion of oxalosuccinic acid to á-ketoglutaric acid

Biotin enzymes are important in protein synthesis, amino acid deamination, purine synthesis and nucleic acid metabolism.

Requirements: Biotin is synthesized by many different microorganisms and certain fungi.

Animal	Requirement
Beef cattle, Dairy cattle, Sheep, Goat, Horse	Microbial synthesis
Cattle calf	10 µg/Kg body weight
Chicken	0.15-0.20 mg/Kg
Swine	0.15-0.20 mg/ Kg
Human	40-200 µg/ day

Sources: Yeast, milk, cereals and vegetables state, pea nuts and eggs.

Food or Feed stuff	Biotin level (μg/gram)
Alfaalfa meal dehydrated	0.33
Corn	0.05-0.20
Peanut	1.63
Soybean meal	0.18-0.50
Eggs whole	0.25
Liver, beef	1.00

Deficiency symptoms: Biotin deficiency is more prevalent in swine and poultry than farm animals. Biotin deficiency could be introduced by giving animal avidin, a protein in raw egg white, which combined with biotin and prevent it absorption from the intestine. The deficiency symptoms are retarded growth and development, falling of hairs (alopecia) and dermatitis characterized by dryness, roughness and brownish exudates, ulceration of skin, transverse of soles and tops of hooves. Recently it has been demonstrated that biotin deficiency is the chief cause of fatty liver and kidney syndrome (FLKS) which is characterized by a lethargic with death. Reduced growth rate, disturbed and broken feathering, dermatitis, leg and weak deformities are observed in poultry.

Choline: It is discovered as an essential part of the phospholipid lecithin. The requirement of the choline is met through two ways (1) By ration (2) By the process of transmethylation. Choline can be synthesized in the liver from methionine. The chemical structure of choline is given below.

$$CH_3 \diagdown \qquad OH$$
$$CH_3 \text{———} N$$
$$CH_3 \diagup \qquad CH_2 \, CH_2OH$$

Functions:

1. Choline is a metabolic essential for building and maintaining cell structure. As a phospholipid it is a structural part of lecithin (phosphatidylcholine), certain plasmalogens and the sphingomyelins.

2. It plays an essential role in fat metabolism in the liver. It prevents abnormal accumulation of fat (fatty liver) by promoting its transport as lecithin or by increasing the utilization of fatty acids in the liver itself. Thus choline is referred as lipotropic factor.

3. It is essential for the formation of acetylchoiline, which is important in the transmission of nerve impulses.

4. Choline is as a source of three labile methyl groups for formation of methionine by the transmethylation reactions.

Deficiency symptoms: Deficiency of choline causes a deficiency of phospholipid in tissues, which are generally concerned with the transportation and oxidation of fatty acid in the liver. As a consequence, fat accumulates in the liver causing fatty liver. So choline is also concerned with the prevention of perosis or sleeped tendon in chicks.

Sources: Natural fat is a good source of choline. Green leafy materials, yeast, egg yolk and cereals are rich sources.

Vitamin-B_{12} (Cyanocobalmin): Rickes and his associates (1948) isolated this vitamin from the liver as pinkish crystalline substance and name it B_{12}. It was also known as animal protein (APF) and antipernicious anaemia factor (APA). In patients suffering from pernicious anaemia the absorption of B_{12} from the gastro intestinal tracts is impaired owing to the absence of a specific glycoprotein termed the "Intrinsic factor" normally secreted in the gastric juice. Vitamin B_{12} has been isolated in several different biologically active forms. Cyanocobalamin, the principle form of the vitamincontains a cyanide group attached to the central cobalt. The cyanide ion may be replaced by a variety of anions *e.g.*, hydroxyl (Hydroxy cobalamin) or nitrite (nitro cobalamin. The biological actions of these derivatives appear to be similar to that of cobalamin. Vitamin B_{12} was the last vitamin to be discovered and the most potent of the vitamin. Vitamin B_{12} is unique that it is synthesized in nature only by the microorganisms.

Absorption and metabolism of vitamin B_{12}: Ingested vitamin B_{12} has to be combined with intrinsic factor produced by the stomach before it can be absorbed. Vitamin is absorbed from terminal ileum leaving the intrinsic factor behind, in the absence of intrinsic factor there is only minimal absorption of the vitamin by passive diffusion. The metabolic role of vitamin B_{12} is associated with availability of tetrahydrofolate and metabolism of some fatty acids.

Functions:

1. There is a nutritional inter-relationship with folic acid, B_{12} vitamin and the metabolism of one-carbon compound.

2. Cobamide coenzyme plays an important role in the transformation of methly malonyl coenyme A to succinyl coenzyme A in the metabolism of propionic acid in ruminats.

3. Vitamin B_{12} and folic acid are required for the formation of DNA whereas vitamin B_{12} alone being necessary for the synthesis of RNA.

4. Folic acid and B_{12} are essential for the maturation of R.B.C. Vitamin B_{12} is necessary in reduction of one carbon compounds of formate and formaldehyde, it participate with folacin in biosynthesis of labile methyl groups. Formation of labile methyl groups is necessary for biosynthesis of purine and pyrimidine bases.

Requirements:

Animal	Requirement
Ruminants, Horse, Rabbit	Microbial synthesis
Cattle calf	0.34-0.68 µg/Kg body weight
Chicken	3-9 µg/Kg
Swine	5-15 µg/Kg
Dog	26 µg/Kg
Human	0.5-4.0 µg/day

Sources: The origin of Vitamin B_{12} in nature appears to be microbial synthesis. Foods of animal origin are good sources i.e. meat, kidney, liver, milk, egg, fish, root nodules of certain legumes contain small quantities of Vitamin B_{12}. It is mostly deficient in grains and fodder crops.

161

Food and food stuffs	Vitamin B_{12} (ppm)
Blood meal	50
Fish meal	130-160
Meat meal	70
Liver meal	540
Milk	54

Deficiency symptoms:

Human: Vitamin B_{12} deficiency causes pernicious anaemia.

Poultry: In poultry, poor growth, poor feathering and kidney damage may occur. In adults hatchability goes down.

Pig: Young pig shows poor growth, show in coordination of the hind legs. Adult pigs show dermatitis, a rough coat, and suboptimal growth.

Ruminants: It has been shown that when the vitamin is deficient, propionic acid can not be metabilized adequately when sufficient cobalt is present in the diet, the sufficient amount of vitamin B_{12} can be synthesized by the rumen microorganism to meet the animal needs.

Vitamin-C (Ascorbic Acid): The name of vitamin C became quite popular in 18th century when it was found that sailors developed a disease called scurvy after they had been at sea for a period of 4 to 5 months. A British Naval Surgeon Dr. Lind in 1747 told that scurvy disease can be prevented by feeding the juice of citrus fruits in human beings. On this basis it was discovered as an Anti- scurvy factor. It was first isolated in 1932 by American scientist King and Hungarian scientist S. Gyorgy. Vitamin C is chemically known as L- ascorbic acid and has the following formula.

The vitamin is colourless, crystalline, water soluble compound having acidic and strong reducing properties. In some species it is synthesized from glucose, via glucuronic acid and gulonic acid lactone; the enzyme L-gulonolactone oxidase is required for the synthesis. Glycoascorbic acid acts as an antimetabolite for vitamin C. This enzyme is absent in guinea

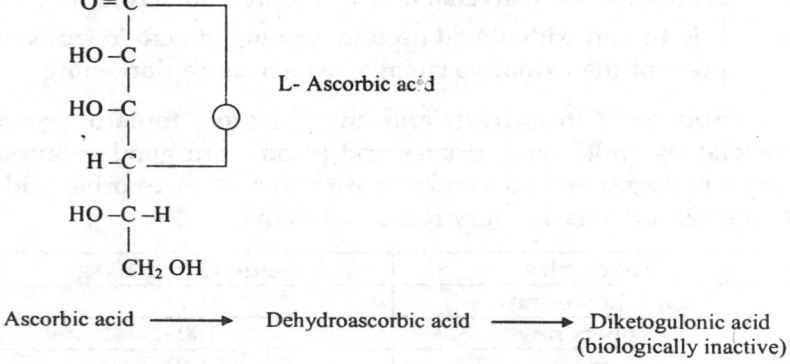

Ascorbic acid ⟶ Dehydroascorbic acid ⟶ Diketogulonic acid
(biologically inactive)

pig, human, bats, certain birds and fishes. Glycoascorbic acid acts as antimetabolites for vitamin-C. One I.U. is the activity of 0.05 mg of ascorbic acid.

Absorption and metabolism: Both forms of vitamin are readily absorbed by active transport and passive diffusion. Vitamin C is absorbed from the small intestine and excreted via urine. There is particularly no storage of this vitamin and secreted in the milk of lactating animals.

Functions:

1. Vitamin C is essential for collagen formation.
2. It aids for the conversion of folic acid to its active form tetrahydrofolic acid.
3. Vitamin C is also involved in the hydroxylation of proline, lysine and aniline, which are important for normal physiology of the animals.
4. It aids iron to stay in reduced state, which is very important tor the body and have stimulatory effect on phagocytic activity of leucocytes.
5. It participates in the synthesis of steroid hormones by the adernal cortex.
6. It involves in the metabolism of lipids, as blood cholesterol level appear to fall with the administration of ascorbic acid and rise due to deficiency of this vitamin.

7. It aids for the conversion of tryptophan to serotonin.

8. It is an antioxidant and used in canning of certain fruits to prevent the oxidative changes which cause darkening.

Sources: Citurs fruits and juices, lemon, tomato, green vegetables, milk, body tissues and plasma are good sources. Dry roughages and concentrates are deficient in ascorbic acid. Guava and Aonla are very rich in vitamin C.

Vegetables	Vitamin C (mg/100 g)
Cauliflower raw	50-90
Peppers raw	100
Spinach	10-60
Corn	12
Potato	8-18
Fruits	10-30
Apple	35-45
Grapes	300
Guavas	80
Lemon	250
Limes	40-60
Orange	40-90
Straw berries	5-30
Fish	3-7

Deficiency symptoms: Man, monkey and guinea pig suffer with severe deficiency of vitamin C is called scurvy. The disease is characterized by weakness, swollen and tenderness of joints, delayed healing of wounds, spongy haemorrhagic friable gum, loose teeth and small haemorrhage which may appear anywhere throughout the body, particularly near the bone and joints and under the skin and mucous membrane due to increase fragility of the blood capillaries. Resistance to infection is reduced. Symptoms of oedema, emaciation and diarrhoea are also appeared.

Unidentified vitamins: The discovery of vitamins is of course a very great research in the field of nutrition. If all the vitamins discovered so far are included in the ration of poultry, even then they may lack in proper development. When these birds are offered fish meal, penicillium mycelium meal, molasses, green leaves and dried skimmed milk. They have a better growth and development. It clearly indicates that these substances contain certain nutrients which are still to be identified. Hence they were called as unidentified viatmins or growth factors. Certain factors which appear to be of some significance in poultry nutrition are the grass factor, whey factor and fish factor. The evidence for these has been obtained from growth responses in feeding trials and from hatchability studies.

Hypervitaminosis: It is the name given to pathological conditions resulting from an overdose of vitamins. In natural conditions, it is unlikely to occur, until the synthetic vitamins are not added in the ration. Clinical sign of hypervitaminosis A in young chicks include loss of appetite, poor growth, diarrhoea, encrustation around the mouth and reddening of the eyelids. In pigs rough coat, Scaly skin, hyperirritability, haemorrhages, periodic termors and even death. Excessive intakes of vitamin D cause abnormally high levels of calcium and phosphorus in the blood, which result in the deposition of calcium and phosphorus in the blood, which result in the deposition of calcium salts in the arteries and organs. Hypervitaminosis K showed a depression in growth and anaemia as toxic symptoms.

Specific deficiency of vitamins:

Vit A: Night blindness, Xerophthalmia
Vit D: Ricket, Osteomalacia
Vit E: White muscle disease (stiff lamb disease), Crazy chick disease, Muscular dystrophy
Vit K: Sweet clover poisoning
Vit C: Scurvy
Thiamine: Beri-beri, Stargazing in poultry
Riboflavin: Curled toe paralysis
Niacin: Black tongue (poultry), Pig pellagra
Pyridoxine: Goose stepping in pig
Pantothenic acid: Goose stepping in pig, Fatty liver in poultry
Biotin: Alopecia, Fatty liver and kidney syndrome (FLKS)
Folic acid: Anaemia
Cyanocobalmin: Pernicious anaemia

Q.1. Fill in the blank.

1. – – – gave the term vitamins
2. Vitamin A was discovered by – – – – – – –.
3. The forms of viatmin A is – – – – – and – – – – –.
4. One International unit of vitamin A is equal to – – – – –-
5. The precursor of vitamin A is – – – – – – –.
6. Anti infective vitamin is – – – – – – –.
7. Vitamin D as an antirachitic factor was discovered by – – – – –.
8. The active forms of vitamin D are – – – – and – – – – –.
9. The precursor of ergocalciferol is – – – – – – –.
10. The precursor of cholecalciferol is – – – – – –.
11. One International unit of vitamin D is equal to – – – – – –.
12. Vitamin D deficiency in young animals is – – – –.
13. In adult animals vitamin D deficiency is – – – – –.
14. The chemical name of vitamin E is – – – – – – –.
15. Vitamin E was discovered by – – – – – – –.
16. Vitamin E and – – – – – enzyme acts as biological anti-oxidant.
17. Stiff lamb disease is caused by – – – – – –.
18. Mulberry heart disease is deficiency symptoms of – – – –.
19. Crazy chick disease is caused by – – – – – –.
20. Exudative diathesis in chicks is deficiency symptoms of – – –.
21. Vitamin K was identified by – – – – –.
22. The naturally occuring form of vitamin K is – – – – and – – – –.
23. Sweet clover poisoning is deficiency symptoms of – – – –.
24. Beri-beri disease is caused by – – – – –.

25. Peripheral polynuritis is deficiency symptoms of — — —.
26. Curled toe paralysis is deficiency symptoms of — — — —.
27. The deficiency symptom of niacin is — — — — in dog.
28. Niacin is prosthetic group in co-enzymes namely — — — — and — — —.
29. Niacin deficiency in pig is known as — — — — — —.
30. Black tenque in poultry is a deficiency symptoms of — — — —.
31. Niacin in body can be synthesized from — — — —.
32. Goose stepping in pig is deficiency symptoms of — — —.
33. The active form of vitamin folic acid is — — — — — —.
34. Perosis in poultry is deficiency symptoms of — — — — — —.
35. Biotin is a prosthetic group in enzymes namely — — — and — — — — —-
36. Deficiency symptoms of biotin is — — — — — —.
37. Choline is an essential part of phospholipid known as — — — —.
38. Deficiency symptoms of choline is — — — — — —-
39. The deficiency symptom of cyanocobalamin is — — — — —.
40. The chemical name of vitamin C is — — — — — — —.
41. The deficiency symptom of vitamin C is — — — — —.

Q.2. Explain the following:

1. Differentiate the fat soluble and water soluble vitamins
2. Define the vitamin.
3. Role of vitamin A in eye – vision.
4. Metabolism of vitamin D.
5. Deficiency symptoms of vitamin E.
6. Role of vitamin K in blood clotting
7. Deficiency symptoms and source of vitamin C.
8. Explain the deficiency symptoms of riboflavin and thiamin

9. Explain the functions and deficiency symptoms of niacin and pyridoxine.
10. Deficiency symptoms of pantothenic acid and folic acid.
11. Functions and deficiency symptoms of biotin and choline.
12. Functions and deficiency symptoms of cyanocobolamin.
13. Write a note on unidentified factor and Hypervitaminosis.
14. Construct tables to compare common features (i.e. functions, sources, sign of deficiency etc.) of the following pairs of vitamins:
    (a) Riboflavin and niacin
    (b) Vitamin B_{12} and folate
    (c) Vitamin C and Vitamin E
    (d) Vitamin D and Vitamin A

Chapter 9

Feed Additives in
Animal Nutrition

Definition of feed additives: Feed additive is an ingredient or combination of ingredients added to the basic feed mix or parts thereof to fulfill the specific need or any chemical incorporated in an animal feed for the purpose of improving rate of gain, feed efficiency or prevention and control of disease. These are used in microquantities and require careful handling and mixing. A feed additive is need not be a drug. Feed additives are of two types.

1. Nutrient feed additives like minerals and vitamin supplements

2. Non-nutrient feed additives like antibiotics, antioxidants, coccidiostat and feed preservatives etc.

Feed additives increase feed quality and feed palatability and improve the animal performance as feed additives are mixed with feeds in non therapeutic quantities for the purpose of promoting animal growth, lowering feed consumption and protecting the animal against all sorts of harmful environmental stresses. Addition of antioxidants to diet produces grades of meat in which the fat does not rancidify or does so more slowly. So the use of additives also makes end products more homogenous and of better quality. Low levels of additives, mainly of antibiotics or other growth promoters and related compounds in animal feed contribute to increase production of animal protein for human consumption so decrease the cost of animal products. Non-nutrient feed additives not classified under nutrients, but are considered as feed supplements.

1. Antibiotic feed supplement: Antibiotic are a group of soluble organic substances produced from microorganism, which in small concentration have the capacity of inhibiting the growth of other microorganism, and even of destroying them. They have the properties of inhibiting at low concentrations for growth, activity or multiplication of other microorganism.

Mode of action of antibiotic:

1. Antibiotic spares protein, amino acid and vitamins.

2. They act by increasing the absorption of B- complex vitamin in gastro- intestinal tract.

3. They increase the absorptive capacity of the intestine.

4. Suppressing or destoying organisms,which produced subclinical infections and compete with the host for supplies of nutrients.

5. Stimulating the growth of microorganism, which synthesizes essential nutrients.

6. Antibiotic alters intestinal bacteria so that less urease is produced and thus less ammonia is formed. As ammonia is harmful and suppresses growth in non-ruminants.

Antibiotics in pig feeding: The good effect of feeding the antibiotic feed supplement is observed with animals given all vegetable protein diets than those receiving animal protein supplements. The increase in growth rate may between 10-20 percent and reducing the feed intake by about 2.5 percent. Highest the nutritive value of ration, the less would be the improvement in growth rate on antibiotic feeding. The antibiotic improves the efficiency of feed utilization to the extent of 5-8 percent. A mixture of two or more antibiotic is no more effective than the single effective antibiotic. The greatest beneficial effect of antibiotic feeding is observed during the early growth period between weaning and 50 Kg body weight, there after the effect diminishes with age. If the antibiotics are stopped in the ration of pigs after 50 Kg body weight, the initial advantage in the improvement of growth rate is last. Therefore, it is recommended to feed the antibiotics till the pigs reach the market weight. Runty pigs give better response with antibiotic feeding. The optimum level for most antibiotics in the diet is within the range 5-15 mg per kg and there is no advantage in exceeding these low levels.

Antibiotics used as feed additives for growth promotion:

Products	Animal dose	(mg/lb. feed)
Bacitracin and derivatives	Poultry	2-25
	Swine	5-25
	Beef	17-35 mg/day
Chlorteracycline	Poultry	5-25
	Swine	5-25
	Beef	25-70 mg/day
Dynafac	Poultry	45-90
	Swine	200 mg/d
	Beef	200 mg/d
	Sheep	300-400 mg/d
Erythromycin	Growing chicks	2.3g.
	Beef	37.0 mg/d
	Poultry	3.5-5.0
	Swine	75.0
Oleandomycin	Broiler and Turkey	0.5-1.0
Oxyretracycline	Poultry	2.5
	Swine	12.25
	Beef	25.75
	Sheep	5-10
Pencillin	Poultry	1.2-25 mg/d
	Swine	5.25
Roxarsone	Poultry	11-22
	Swine	11-33
Tyrosin	Poultry	2-25
	Swine	5-25

Source. Animal nutrition growth by Hafez and Dyer (1969).

Antibiotics in Poultry feeding: Pencillin is more effective than other antibiotics especially to young and growing chicks. It increases the growth rate and this effect is most marked upto one month of age. As with pigs, the effect diminishes with age.

171

The highest effect is upto 6 weeks of age. In the laying birds the egg production is also improved. About 5 g of procaine pencillin per ton of ration for poultry is needed; but to control diseases, a higher level of 50 gm or more/ton for feed is used. Use of a combination of antibiotics has been no more effective than that of single effective antibiotic. In layer, egg production has not been increased by adding antibiotics to a ration which is nutritionally complete. But, if hens are fed on only vegetables product ration, an antibiotic vitamin B_{12} feed supplement may increase both egg production and hatchability.

Antibiotic in ruminant feeding: The addition of antibiotics supplement in calf rations has increased the growth rate of dairy calves specially when there had been much trouble from disease in the herd. It has reduced the incidence of scours and other infectious disease. Most of the growth improvement occurs before up to 8-10 weeks of age at the rate of 30 mg of Auromycin or Terramycin per calf daily. As far as adult animals are concerned, the results are conflicting. It has been assumed that the inclusion of antibiotics in the diet could be harmful by suppressing the activity of cellulotytic organisms and thus impairing cellulose digestion and other rumen microorganisms are also depressed. So feeding antibiotics after 12 weeks of age has not beneficial effect on the animals. Following points should be kept in mind while using antibiotics for animal feeding.

1. Antibiotics should be used only for:

    a. Growing and fattening pigs

    b. Growing chicks and turkey

    c. Growing calves upto the age of 10-12 weeks.

2. Antibiotics should not be used in the feed of ruminant animals breeding pigs and breeding and laying poultry stock.

3. While adding antibiotics at the recommended level, care should be taken that they are thoroughly and evenly mixed with the feed.

4. For the best result, antibiotics should be used with properly balanced feeds.

5. Antibiotics are not a substitute for good management and healthy living condition or for properly balanced ration.

Antibiotics feeding hazards in animals: There has been a serious concern about the indiscriminate use of antibiotics as feed supplement in the animals. The meat from these animals contains the residue of the antibiotics and constant use by the human being could present a hazard to human health because of the potential development of enteric bacteria.

2. Hormones: Some of the hormones used as a growth promoting agents in livestock such as estrogens, androgens, progesterone, growth hormones, thyroxin and thyroproteins. Iodinated casein is a commercial product which has given variable response. This compound has been given response for a shorter period in the lactating animals. Long term feeding gave discouraging results.

The growth promoting hormones are grouped into two on the basis of their effects on the body.
1. Anabolic: (Somatotropin, thyroxin and androgens)
2. Catabolic (estrogen and glucocorticoids)

1. Anabolic agents: The hormones of the anabolic class by nature exert their effect on both skeleton and protein metabolism. Somatotrapin stimulates growth of endochondral bones and epiphysis of long bones while in protein metabolism it aids nitrogen and overall protein synthesis. Thyroxin also stimulates growth of long bones as well as protein synthesis. Testosterone at low dose increases the epiphyseal diameter, promotes muscles growth by angmenting nitrogen retention.

2. Catabolic agent: The hormone belonging to catabolic group similarly exert their on both skeleton and protein metabolism. Estrogen inhibits skeletal growth although in ruminants it increases nitrogen retention. Gluco corticoids decrease growth of epiphysis and also aid in degrading protein and amino acids and there by inhibit protein synthesis in extrahepatic tissues.

Effect of hormones on milk production: It is an established fact that milk production in the cow will increase following the feeding of thyroprotein or thyroxine. The most effective daily dose appears to be about 15 g/cow in case of thyroprotein and 100mg/cow daily for thyroxine. The addition of hormones in the diet of cows has increase milk production from 15 to 20% above control animals, if concomitant increase in energy intake was maintained. If additional feed is not given then the response is either very poor or nill.

Effect of hormone on growth: Synthetic oestrogenic hormones like stilbesterol are being used in many countries as growth promoters. Studies with fattening lambs have shown that feeding 2-5 mg of stilbesterol daily increase the average daily gain about 20 percent and reduced the feed Intake per unit of gain. These substances either be given at the rate of 10 mg/day in beef cattle or can be implanted under the skin in the form of pellets in a single dose of 75 g and 10 mg in sheep. Synthetic estrogens should never be given to female animals; otherwise there will be derangement of the breeding behaviour. Some workers have reported increased rate of gain improved feed efficiency as a results of feeding thyroprotein or thyroxin to growing pigs from the time of weaning to market weight.

Harmful effect of hormone feeding:

1. There are certain side effects in the animals fed on synthetic hormones, such as (a) restlessness (b) milk secretion from rudimentary teats etc.

2. The most serious danger is to the human being arising from the residues of synthetics estrogen in the meat which have carcinogenic properties.

3. Feeding of thyroprotein in dairy animals causes general excitability and injuries in the body.

Optimal amount of oral dose or implantation of various hormonal compounds as reported by the National Research Council Committee are given below.

Hormones and their doses for livestock:

Products	Animals	Doses	Method of use
Diethylstilbestrol	Cattle	10mg/d	In feed mash
	Sheep	2mg/d	In feed mash
Thyroprotein	Cattle	24 to36mg	Subcutaneous
	Poultry	12 to15mg	Subcutaneous
Diethylstilbesterol + testosterone	Cattle	24mg + 120mg	Subcutaneous
Thiouracil	Swine and poultry	0.2 percent of diet	In feed mash
Iodinated casein (thyroprotein)	Lactating cow	200mh/kg diet	In feed mash
	Lactating cow	25-5 mg/kg diet	In feed mash

3. Probiotics: The term probiotic means 'for life'. These are live cultures of non-pathogenic viable organisms which are administered orally. Probiotics are coined by Parker in 1974 as an organisms and substances which contribute to intestinal microbial balance. Fuller in 1989 defined probiotics as live microbial feed supplements which beneficially affect the host animal by improving its intestinal microbial balance. Probiotics are available in pastes, powder and liquid form or directly fed feed additives. The term pronutrient may also be used for probiotic. Most commonly used microorganisms, as probiotics are *Lactobacillus acidophillus, Lactobacillus fermentum, Lactobacillus lactis, Aspergillus oryzae, Streptococcus* foecium, *Saccharomyces cerevisiae* etc. Live yeast culture, Direct fed microbials (DFM) and curds are examples of probiotics

Characteristics of a good probiotics:

1. It should not be toxic or pathogenic to the host.

2. It should have a positive effect on the host.

3. It should be posses high survival rate and multiply faster in the digestive tract. The adhesive capability to micro organisms must be firm and faster.

4. It should be cheap and economical.

5. Feeding of probiotics to animals should be easy, safe and simple.

4. Prebiotics: Prebiotics are non-digestible feed ingredients that beneficially affect the host by selectively stimulating the growth and or activity of one or limited number of bacteria in the colon that can improve the host health. Galacto oligosaccharides, fructooligosaccharides and lactose derivatives have been used in poultry and other non-ruminants. Oligosaccharides may directly inhibit the growth of certain intestinal pathogenic species by increasing the concentration of lactic acid which will decrease the pH in the lower gut Microbes are able to attach themselves to the mucosa through recognition of oligosaccharide binding sites on the wall. Dietary oligosaccharides attract microbes away from the intestinal binding sites and therefore, reducing colonization of pathogens. Chicken treated with caeca (Bailey *et al.*, 1991) and the reduction was attributed to shift in the intestinal gut microflora. More over, certain oligosaccharides like a-1,2- gluco oligosaccharides substrate for beneficial *Bifidobacterium sp.* at lower tract which favoured their colonization and prevent colonization of harmful bacteria.

5. Arsenicals: It was reported that organic arsenals had growth promoting properties similar to those of antibiotics when added to the diet of chicks. In addition to their use as growth stimulants, these have been used at low levels to help protect feeds from microbial destruction and to prevent and control poultry diseases. Arsanilic acid, sodium arsanilate are compounds used.

6. Tranquilizers: A number of tranquilizing drugs have been usually used to combat stress due to heat or other environmental factors. Certain tranquilizers such as natural alkaloid of Rauwolfia, reserpine, hydroxyzine, chloropromazine have been shown in certain trails to improve daily live weight gain to livestock. The compounds act by reducing hypertension and nervousness specially in summer or under any stress condition.

7. Copper sulphate: At 0.1 percent level of the diet in fattening pigs, improve the rate of gain and feed conversion efficiency between weaning and bacon weight. Sheep are particularly susceptible to copper poisoning, and there are several instances of death through sheep eating copper fortified pigmeals.

8. Anthelmentics, coccidiostat and antifungal: Anthelmentics are the deworming drugs and used periodically in the feed or water to prevent parasitic infestation, specially of round warm. Out of many commercial products, 2,2 dichlorovinyl dimethyl phosphate, has both anthelmintics and separate growth stimulatory effect in cattle. Coccidiostat are routinely used in the diets of the poultry to prevent the most devastating type of disease the coccidiosis. Antifungals are natural or synthetic substances which inhibit the growth of fungi.

9. Pigmenters and flavoring agents: Pigmenters are usually carotenoid sources added to feed to improve pigmentation of broilers and egg yolk. Some time some flavouring substances are also used as feed additives to improve the palatability of certain feed stuffs.

10. Antioxidants: Fats are subject to oxidation with development of rancidity, which reduces palatability, and may cause some digestive and nutritional problems. Antioxidants are added for the stabilization of fats and fat soluble vitamins and also to prevent the destruction of vitamin by oxidation. Vitamin E is a good antioxidant of vitamin A, carotene and fats. The antioxidants which are recommended to prevent rancidity of fat are DPPD (Diphenyl-para-phenylene-diamine), BHA (Butylated hydroxy anisole), BHT (Butylated hydroxy toluene) and ethoxwuin.

Q1. Fill in the blanks.

1. Antibiotic feed additives are recommended in animals like – – – and – –.

2. – – – – and – – – – are most commonly used antibiotics feed additives.

3. In ruminants antibiotics feed additives are used at a age upto – – – –.

4. — — — and — — — — are catabolic hormones used as feed additives.

5. — — — — and — — — — are anabolic hormones used as feed additives.

6. Feeding of hormone — — — — — the milk production.

7. — — — — and — — — — are the side effects of hormones feed additives.

8. — — — — and — — — — are hormones used as feed additives.

9. — — — — and — — — — — are bacteria used as probiotics.

10. The term probiotics are coined by — — — — — — — —.

11. Examples of probiotics are — — — — and — — — — — —.

12. Copper sulphate is used as feed additive in pig at a rate of — — — — — —.

Q.2. Explain the following.

1. Antibiotics feeding in non-ruminants.

2. Probiotics as a feed additive.

3. Mode of action of antibiotics as feed additives.

4. Harmful effect of antibiotic feeding.

5. Harmful effect of hormone feeding

6. Pigmenters and flavouring agents as feed additives.

PART-II

Course No. ANN- 212
(Evaluation of feed stuffs and feed technology)

Chapter 1

Classification of Common Feeds and Fodders

The animals are dependent on plants for the supply of their food material. They consume forage, straws, concentrates and their byproducts for various body functions. These feed stuffs can be grouped as roughages and concentrates on the basis of bulkiness and chemical composition (Table 1).

1. Roughages: These are the feed stuffs which contain more than 18% crude fibre and less than 60% TDN and more than 35% cell wall on dry matter basis. These are further subdivided into following ways.

A. On the basis of nutrient density:

1. **Maintenance type roughages:** They have 3-5 percent DCP and fed to animals as a maintenance ration. Examples are green maize, sorghum and oat etc.

2. **Non-maintenance type roughages:** They have below 3% DCP and can not provide maintenance ration to animals when fed alone. Examples are straw, stover and kadbi etc.

3. **Productive type roughages:** They provide production ration to the animals and have 3-5 percent DCP. Examples are berseem, lucerne and cowpea etc.

B. On the basis of the season of cultivation:

1. **Kharif roughage:** These are grown during the period of June to October. Examples are cowpea, guar, rice, bean, bajra, jowar, maize and teosinte etc.

2. **Rabi crops:** These are grown from October to March month of the year. Examples are berseem, lucerne, mentha, sarson, oat, barley etc.

Table 1: Classification of feeds and fodders

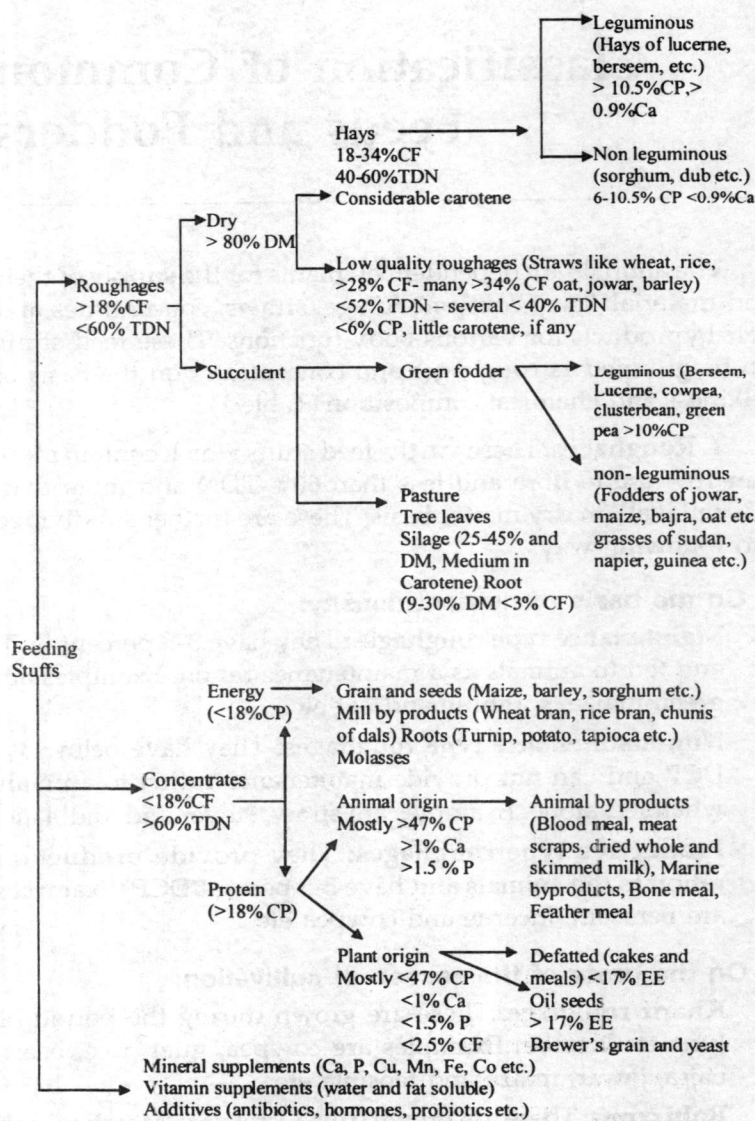

Feeding Stuffs

Roughages
>18%CF
<60% TDN

Dry
> 80% DM

Hays
18-34%CF
40-60%TDN
Considerable carotene

Leguminous
(Hays of lucerne,
berseem, etc.)
> 10.5%CP,>
0.9%Ca

Non leguminous
(sorghum, dub etc.)
6-10.5% CP <0.9%Ca

Low quality roughages (Straws like wheat, rice,
>28% CF- many >34% CF oat, jowar, barley)
<52% TDN – several < 40% TDN
<6% CP, little carotene, if any

Succulent

Green fodder

Leguminous (Berseem,
Lucerne, cowpea,
clusterbean, green
pea >10%CP

non- leguminous
(Fodders of jowar,
maize, bajra, oat etc.
grasses of sudan,
napier, guinea etc.)

Pasture
Tree leaves
Silage (25-45% and
DM, Medium in
Carotene) Root
(9-30% DM <3% CF)

Concentrates
<18%CF
>60%TDN

Energy
(<18%CP)

Grain and seeds (Maize, barley, sorghum etc.)
Mill by products (Wheat bran, rice bran, chunis
of dals) Roots (Turnip, potato, tapioca etc.)
Molasses

Protein
(>18% CP)

Animal origin
Mostly >47% CP
>1% Ca
>1.5 % P

Animal by products
(Blood meal, meat
scraps, dried whole and
skimmed milk), Marine
byproducts, Bone meal,
Feather meal

Plant origin
Mostly <47% CP
<1% Ca
<1.5% P
<2.5% CF

Defatted (cakes and
meals) <17% EE
Oil seeds
> 17% EE
Brewer's grain and yeast

Mineral supplements (Ca, P, Cu, Mn, Fe, Co etc.)
Vitamin supplements (water and fat soluble)
Additives (antibiotics, hormones, probiotics etc.)

3. **Zaid roughages:** These are grown in summer season from April to June. Examples are cow pea, guar, maize, bajra etc.

C. On the basis of legumes:

1. **Leguminous roughage:** These are roughages having dicotyledons seed and rich in protein i.e. berseem, lucerne, cowpea etc.

2. **Non-leguminous roughage:** The roughages having monocotyledon seeds are called non-leguminous roughages i.e. bajra, maize, oat, barley etc.

Stage of Plant Growth: Stage of Maturity is an important factor that influences the nutritive value of forages, silages. In perennial fodders the actual growing time of plant is used as stage of maturity.

i. **Early vegetative:** Stage at which the plant is vegetative and before the stem elongates.

ii. **Late vegetative:** Stage at which stems are beginning to elongate just before blooming, first bud to first flower.

iii. **Early bloom:** Stage between initiation of bloom and stage in which $1/_{10}$ of the plants are in bloom.

iv. **Mid-bloom:** $1/_{10}$ to $2/_{3}$ of the plants are in bloom.

v. **Late-bloom:** Stage in which blossoms begin to dry and fall and seeds begin to form.

vi. **Milk Stage:** Seeds well formed, soft & immature.

vii. **Dough stage:** Seeds with dough like consistency.

viii. **Mature:** Stage at which plant is harvested for seeds.

ix. **Past ripe:** Stage that follows maturity.

Non Leguminous fodder:

Maize (*Zea mays*): This crop is very much popular among the farmers due to it's dual use for grains as well as fodder. Maize forage is more nutritious at milk stage. It is non-leguminous kharif crop. It is a maintenance type fodder having 8-10 per cent protein.

Jowar/Sorghum (*Sorghum vulgare*): It is also non-leguminous kharif crop grown under irrigated and non-irrigated conditions. For feeding of livestock it should be harvested at 50% flowering stage of growth. Green jowar contains 0.5 % DCP, 16% TDN, 0.13% calcium and 0.03% phosphorus.

Bajra or Pearl Millet (*Pennesetum typhoids*): It is grown as a grain crop. But when grown for fodder crop, it is harvested before flowering stage for feeding the animals. It contains 13% TDN and 0.9% DCP.

Teosinte or Mak Chari: It is an inter-genetic cross between maize and chari and grown in those areas which are suitable for maize and chari. It contains 6.0% DCP and 55% TDN on dry matter basis.

Oats (*Avena sativa*): This is a non-leguminous crop of the rabi season. It is the best crop for haymaking. It is a maintenance type fodder having 7-9 percent CP and 55% TDN.

Leguminous fodder:

Berseem (*Trifolium alexandrium*): Berseem is one of the most important cultivated forage crops of India. Kashni is the weed crop grown along with berseem. It is grown in rabi season. It contains 15% CP and 60 % TDN. But excessive intake of berseem may leads to bloat condition.

Senji (*Melilotus parviflora*): It is also an important leguminous rabi crop. It contains 2.5% DCP and 13% TDN on fresh basis.

Lucerne (*Medicago sativa*): This is a productive type fodder which can support growth as well as milk production when fed alone. It contains 12-15 % CP and 55-60% TDN.

Lobia or Cow pea (*Vigna sinensis*): It is one of the most important fodder crops of irrigated land for the summer season. It contains on an average 15% CP and 30% crude fibre on dry matter basis.

Grasses: These are the self grown as well as cultivated plants which are used for grazing animals as well as stall- fed animals. Grasses are available in most of the season of the year. Most commonly cultivated grasses are Pusa giant Napier grass, guinea grass, sudan grass and para grass whereas dub grass and many other grasses as a weed in cultivated crops are self-grown grasses. The grasses have a wide range of nutritive value because of different species, varieties and stage of cutting etc. On an average grasses contain 3-20 percent crude protein, 20-40 percent crude fibre which is inversely related to the protein content, and less than 4 percent lipid. The moisture content is high (75-85 per cent) in early stage of growth and reduces towards maturity. Soluble carbohydrates of pastures contain fructan, glucose, fructose, sucrose and raffinose whereas cellulose and hemicellulose are cell wall components which increase with maturity.

Tree leaves: Tree leaves feeding is a common practice in many parts of India especially for sheep, goat and camel. There is wide variation in nutritive value of tree leaves which ranges upto 20 percent crude protein, 25 percent crude fibre, 5-10 percent ether extract, 10 percent ash material and 40 percent nitrogen free extract. Tree leaves are rich source of calcium and poor source of phosphorus. So these have unbalanced Ca: P ratio. Most of the tree leaves contain tannic acid, which is a toxic factor for animals and reduces the availability of protein so digestibility of protein is reduced. Mimosine is another toxic factor present in tree leaves. Tree leaves are fed as grazing the animals or by making a tree leaf mixture, which is also used as a protein, supplement especially in ruminants. Subabul, pakar, gular, pipal, neem, bargad and casuarina leaves are most commonly used for animal feeding.

Roots and Tubers: The roots include carrots, turnips and sugar beet. The sugar beet is grown primarily for its sugar content and is normally not given to animals as such. However, the two by-products from the sugar extraction industry, sugar beet pulp and molasses are important and nutritionally valuable animals foods. The main tubers are potatoes, tapioca or cassava and sweet potato grown extensively in India.

Roots: The root contains high moisture (75-95 per cent)

and low crude fibre (4-13%). The organic matter of roots consists mainly of sugars (50-75%) and is of high digestibility (80-90%). Roots are generally low in crude protein although like most other crops these components can be influenced by the application of nitrogenous fertilizers.

Carrots (*Daucus carota*): Carrots are not given on a large scale for feeding to farm animals. This crop is mainly grown for human consumption as vegetable, halwa and salad. Even then carrot is a valuable feed for all classes of animal being particularly for horses. Carrot has a dry matter content of about 11-13 per cent and ME value of 12.8 MJ/kg of dry matter. The carrot is a rich source of carotene.

Turnips: Turnip is grown as vegetable crops in India. This can be grown in a variety of soil, including alkaline soil. The root can be fed to animals but in practice it is not common feed for livestock in India. There are two types of trunips that are grown, the yellow fleshed cultivars which have high dry matter content than the white fleshed cultivars. It contains 9.0 percent dry matter, 92.2 percent organic matter, 1.2 percent crude protein, 1.1 percent crude fibre and 72.0 percent digestible organic matter.

Sugar beet: Most sugar beet is grown for commercial sugar production, though it is sometime given to animals, especially cow and pigs. Because of its hardness the beet should be pulped or chopped before feeding. It contains 22-25 percent dry matter, 4-6 percent crude protein, 4-6 percent crude fibre, 65-75 percent sugar. Digestible organic matter is about 85-90 percent whereas digestibility of crude protein is about 35-40 percent. After extraction of the sugar of the sugar beet factory, two valuable by-products are obtained which are given to farm animals. These are sugar beet pulp and molasses.

Sugar beet pulp: After extraction of the sugar from sugar beet the residue is called sugar beet pulp. The water content of this product is 80-85 percent. The sugar beet pulp mainly consists of cell wall polysaccharides and consequently the crude fibre content is relatively high. The crude protein and phosphorus content is low. Beet pulp is extensively used as a feed for dairy cows and is also given to fattening cattle and sheep. It is not suitable for pig and poultry because of high crude fibre content in it. It contains 18 percent dry matter, 96 percent organic matter, 10.6 percent crude protein, 20.6 percent crude fibre and 84 percent digestible organic matter.

Beet molasses: After separation of sugar from the water extract, a thick black liquid remains known as molasses. The product has 70-75 percent dry matter. It contains about 90-95 percent organic matter and 2-4 percent crude protein. Most of the crude protein presents in the forms of non-protein nitrogen compounds, including the amine, betaine, which is responsible for the fishy aroma associated with the extraction processes. Molasses is used, generally at a level of 5-10 per cent of the ration, in the manufacture of feed mash and pellets. The molasses not only improves the palatability of the product but also acts as a binding agent. Since molasses is a rich and relatively cheap source of soluble sugar and it is some times used as an additive in silage making.

Tubers: Tuber differs from root crops in containing either starch or fructans instead of sucrose as the main storage carbohydrates. They have higher dry matter and lower crude fibre contents and are more suitable than roots for feeding to pigs and poultry. The main tubers are potato, tapioca and sweet potato.

Tapioca or Cassava (*Manihot esculenta*): Tapioca is a tuber crop grown in Kerala and parts of Tamilnadu. In Kerala about 0.6 million tonnes of leaves are available at the time of harvest. Cassava is a tropical shrubby perennial plant, which produces tuber at the base of the stem. The chemical composition of these tubers varies with maturity, cultivars and growing conditions. Cassava tubers are used for the production of tapioca starch (*Sabudana*) for human consumption, although the tuber is also given to cattle, pig and poultry. It contains 35-40 percent dry matter, 90-98 percent organic matter, 3.4 percent crude protein and 4.3 percent crude fibre.

The p¹ants and tubers contain certain degree of poison since they contain varying proportion of two cyanogenic glucosides (Linamarin and lotaustralin), which readily break down to give hydrocyanic acid. In all cases care must be taken to use the tuber and plant. It should be used after boiling, grating or squeezing or grinding to a powder and then pressing.

Experiments have been carried out for utilizing tapioca waste as an ingredient of cattle and pig ration. It contains 2 percent DCP and 64 percent TDN on dry matter basis for ruminants. Growth and lactation studies in cattle with tapioca waste, replacing the entire maize protein in concentrate mixture, have shown that it can be used as one of the ingredient of the concentrate mixture.

Potatoes (*Solanum tuberosum*): It differs from the root crops, in that the main component is starch and not sucrose. The starch contents of the dry them particularly suitable for pigs and poultry. The crude fibre content is about 3-4 percent. The crude protein of the dry matter is approximately 9-10 percent, about half of this being in the form of non-protein nitrogenous compounds. The protein of uncooked potatoes is poorly digested.

Potatoes are a poor source of minerals, except of the abundant element potassium, the calcium content being particularly low. The phosphorus content is higher since this element is an integral part of the potato starch molecules, but some 20 percent of it is in the form of phytates.

Sweet potatoes (*Ipomoea batata*): The sweet potato is a very important tropical plant whose tubers are widely grown for human consumption and as a commercial source of starch. The tubers are of similar nutritional value to ordinary potatoes although much higher dry matter and lower crude protein content. It contains 32 percent dry matter, 96-97 percent organic matter, 3.9 percent crude protein and 32.8 percent crude fibre.

Concentrates: Concentrate contains little amount of crude fibre and more than 60% TDN. Concentrates constitute essential part of ration. This is well known fact that roughages alone can not supply all the essential nutrients to the producing, growing and working animals. They include oil seed cakes, cereal grains and their byproducts.

Cereal Grains: The cereal grains are high in starch and low in fibre. They are rich in TDN and net energy. The digestible crude protein ranges between 7-10 percent and TDN from 70-80 percent. Starch occurs in the endosperm of the grain in the form of granule. The cereals are all deficient in calcium containing less than 1g/kg DM. The phosphorus content is higher being 3-5g/kg DM. The cereal grains are deficient in vitamin D. Calves, pigs and poultry depend upon cereal grains for their main source of energy.

Barley (*Hordeum sativum*): Barley being the second main rabi crop of India. It contains 7-8 percent DCP and 75-80 percent TDN, 0.07 percent Ca and 0.28 percent P. Barley is deficient in vitamin A, D and riboflavin but rich in niacin content.

Maize (Zea mays): Maize contains 7 percent DCP and 80 percent TDN. The yellow maize contains enough amount of carotene, hence good for feeding of livestock and poultry birds. Protein content varies from 8-12 percent. It is deficient in lysine and methionine. Maize contains about 730 gm starch/Kg DM, is very low in fibre and has a high metabolised energy value.

Gram: Gram contains 12 to 16 percent DCP and 78 percent TDN. Animals have great liking for this grain and so, used for preparing the concentrate mixture for feeding the livestock.

Jowar: Whole grains are usually fed to chickens. It contains 7 percent DCP and 74 percent TDN and high percentage of leucine. Due to high content of leucine, too much feeding of jowar may result in development of niacin deficiency symptoms – a disease called pellagra.

Bajra: Bajra contain crude protein ranges from 10-12 percent and TDN from 70-75 percent. It can be used in place of maize in swine and poultry feeding.

Oat (*Avena sativa*): The oat has always a favourite cereal for ruminant animals and horses but has been less popular in pig and poultry feeding because of its comparatively high fibre content and low energy value. The crude protein content which ranges from 70-150 g/kg DM. Oat contains 7-9 percent DCP and 70-72 percent TDN. It contains 0.12 percent Ca and 0.33 percent P. It is more palatable and nutritious as compared to other cereal grains.

Wheat: Depending upon variety, the crude protein range from 8-14%. It is good source of energy but is seldom used for livestock feeding in the country. It contains 12-14 percent crude protein and 85 percent TDN Poultry are less susceptible, although wheat with high gluten content should not be given since a doughy mass may accumulate in the crop.

Rice: Rice (*Oryza sativa*) is main cereal crop of eastern and southern Asia. It is good source of energy but is seldom used for livestock feeding. It's byproduct rice polish contain 12-14 percent crude protein and about 12 percent of oil. Rice threshed, has a thick fibrous husk or hull like Oat, the state is known as rough rice. The hull is easily removed to leave product known as brown rice. Rough rice may be used as a food for ruminant and horse but brown rice is preferable for pigs. The hulls are high in fibre content and can contain upto 210 g/kg DM of silica.

Oil seed cakes: These are the by-products left after the extraction of oil from oil seeds. In India oil cakes are prepared by two methods e.g.

(1) Machine made (expeller pressed) (2) Ghani pressed.

Ghani pressed cake is more nutritious as compared to expeller pressed and is widely used by farmer in village for feeding their animals. Special care is needed in preserving these feeds because they are more susceptible to fermentation action and mould growth. According to the method of processing, the cakes can be classified as:

1. Ghani pressed Cake- Contain 10-12 percent ether extract.
2. Expeller pressed cake- It contain 6-8 per cent ether extract.
3. Solvent extracted cake- It contain less than 1 percent ether extract. So also called deoiled cake. But this type of cake

contains more percentage of crude protein than other cakes.

Cotton seed Cakes: In cotton growing area it is main source of protein to livestock. It contains 38-40 percent crude protein and is very much used for feeding of milch cattle. Cake contains 18 percent DCP, 72 percent TDN, 0.11 percent Ca and 0.53 percent P. The cake contains more than 0.065 percent gossypol and deficient in lysine and not fit for feeding to swine, poultry and calves. When upper covering of seed is removed (dehulling) and pressed to form cake than known as decorticated cake which is rich in crude protein and low in crude fibre than undecorticated cake.

Linseed cake: It contains about 26 percent DCP, 72 percent TDN, 0.49 percent Calcium and 0.89 percent P. Linseed cake is very much used for feeding of horse and young calves. It is good for pregnant animals. It is good source of protein for cattle, buffalo, sheep and swine but is not good source of protein in poultry ration. Immature linseed contains a small amount of cyanogenetic glycoside, linamarin and linase enzyme which hydrolysed it into hydrogen cyanide which is very toxic to animals. Normal processing conditions destroy the linase and then cake is safe for feeding. Linseed meal has a protective action against selenium poisoning.

Ground nut cake: It contains 40-50 percent crude protein, 70-75 percent TDN 0.08 percent calcium and 0.23 percent phosphorus. It is an important source of protein for livestock feeding. The content of oil is variable according to process of extraction of oil. It contains 10-12 percent in ghani pressed, 6-8 percent in expeller pressed and 0.5-0.7 percent fat in solvent extracted cake. Groundnut cake is fed to cattle, buffalo, sheep, goat, poultry and swine. It is liable to contain a toxic factor known as aflatoxin (B_1(most toxic), B_2, G_1 and G_2) which is produced by the fungus *Aspergillus flavus* particularly during warm rainy season. It may also be rancid particularly during rainy season. Therefore it should not be stored for more than 6 weeks.

Til cake: It contains enough amounts of calcium, phosphorus, & protein and can be kept preserve for longer period. It contains about 38-40 percent DCP and 75-78 percent TDN. The hulls of sesame seeds contain oxalates and it is essential that meals should be completely decorticated in order to avoid toxicities.

Mustard cake: Widely used cake in India. It is very much used in village for feeding the working buffalo. It contains 34-37 percent crude protein, 27 percent DCP, 65-70 percent TDN, 0.29 percent Ca and 0.39 percent P. In case of poultry and pig it is not a good source of protein. About 10-15 percent of it can be incorporated in poultry and swine ration. It contains glucosinolate which on hydrolysis release goiterogenic substance such as thiocynate and isothiocynate which produce goitre. Goiterogenic compound present in mustard cake reduces the growth rate in poultry and swine.

Coconut cake: In coconut growing area, cake is used for feeding the animals. It contains about 7-10 percent DCP (21 percent crude protein), 8 percent fat, 12 percent crude fibre and 8 percent ash.

Rice bran cake: It is very good feed for feeding the livestock. When it is mixed with some other substances has better nutritive value as cattle feed.

Soyabean cake: Soyabean contains from 160-210 g/kg of oil and are generally solvent extracted. It is generally one of the best sources of protein available to animals. It is poor source of vitamin-B and these must be provided either as a supplement or in the form of an animal protein. If no supplementation sow may produce weak litter and older pigs show in co-ordination and failure to walk.

Neem cake: Neem seed contains about 40-45 percent oil. It contains about 13 percent protein of which about 50-60 percent digestible. It is not palatable. It can be incorporated upto the level of 25 to 30 percent in concentrate mixture.

Rubber seed cake: It is available in fairly large quantities in area where rubber plantations are available. Maximum availability is in Kerala state. It contains 16.6 percent DCP, 78.8 percent TDN for pig where as for cattle it contains 18.6 percent DCP and 54 percent TDN.

Agro-industrial by-products: Various agro-industrials by-products are used as animal feed. These are further divided as:

A- Concentrate By-product:

Wheat bran: It is product obtained after wheat flour is removed from the husk. It is widely used as concentrate mixture for dairy animals. It contains 10 percent DCP, 65 percent TDN, 0.07 percent Ca and 0.35 percent P. In concentrate mixture for growing young calves wheat bran may be incorporated upto 50 percent of total grain mixture.

Rice bran: It is mostly used for horses. Feeding of rice bran alone may result in colic pain due to formation of ball inside the intestine. It contains 7 percent DCP, 65 percent TDN, 0.06 percent calcium and 1.12 percent phosphorus. It is also used for cattle, buffaloes, sheep, swine and poultry feeding.

Rice polish: Rice polish contains about 3 percent fibre, 12 percent fat and 12-14 percent protein. It is excellent source of energy and rich in vitamin B- complex.

Husk or chunies: It is obtained as a by- product during process of pulse making. It contains enough of nutrients and is used for feeding the animal along with the concentrate mixture.

Maize gluten feed: It is obtained after removal of most of starch and germ from maize. Maize gluten meal generally contains 45-48 percent protein.

B-Animal By-product:

Fish meal: Fish meal is produced by cooking fish, and pressing the cooked mass to remove most of the oils and water. It is highly nutritious feed obtained from fish body. It contains about 10 percent moisture, 55 percent protein, 6.9 percent fat and 25 percent mineral salt particularly 5.4 percent Ca and 3.4 percent P. It contains vitamin A, D and richest source of vitamin B_{12}. Sterilized fish meal should be used for feeding animals.

Blood meal: Major slaughter house by-product which contains over 80 percent crude protein, but poor in Ca and P. Blood meal is incorporated only in poultry ration in this country.

Meat meal: This is obtained by boiling and drying the meat obtained from dead animals which is subjected to fine powder. It contains almost all the nutrients found in meat and is rich source of animal protein.

Feathers Meal: Poultry feathers are not digested by single stomach animals. When feathers are processed under low pressures (130^0C, 2 ½ hours) or under high pressures (145^0C, 30 min) and dried at about 60^0C. This product is extremely high in protein but deficient in several essential amino acids. It is used primarily in ration of swine and poultry.

Bone Meal: Bone meal is rich in calcium, phosphorus & low in protein. It is used primarily in rations of swine & poultry.

Sugarcane plant by-products:

Sugarcane by-products are also used as animal feeds which are tabulated as below :

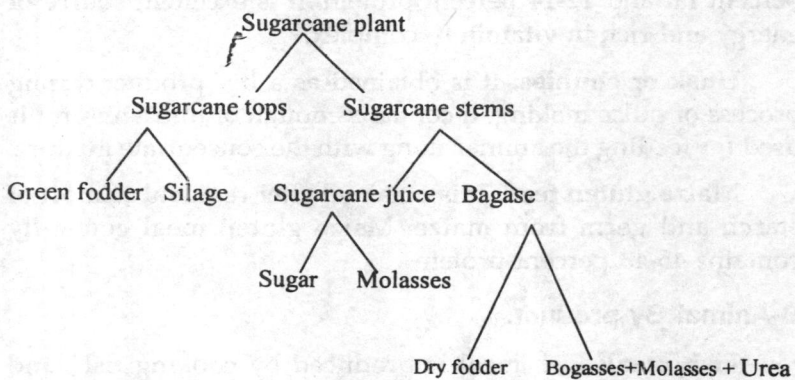

Feed resources availability: Feed resources are broadly classifieds in to three major categories viz. crop residue, concentrates and green fodder. Over the last two decades the total feed resources has increased by 37 percent while the crop residue, concentrate and green fodder have increased by 52, 76 and 2 percent, respectively so efficient management of feed resources would be a vital component in the livestock sector. The growth in feed resources availability especially the concentrate and green fodder have not been commensurate with the increase in the demand of these resources by the livestock.

Dry matter availability at national level (million tonnes)

Feed resources	Years			Required 2004-05	% Deficit
	1985-86	1995-96	2004-05		
Crop residue	240.7	305.1	365.8	412	11
Concentrate	19.6	30.2	34.5	47	28
Green fodder	124.3	124.3	126.6	193	35
Total	384.6	459.6	526.9	652	19

Q.1. Fill in the blanks.

1. Kharif roughages are — — — — — — — and — — — — — — — — — — — — —.

2. The examples of Rabi crops are — — — — — — — — — — and — — — — — — — —.

3. Examples of maintenance type roughages are — — — — — — — — — and — — — — — — which contain — — — — — — — — percent DCP.

4. — — — — — — — — and — — — — — — — — are productive type roughages which contain — — — — — — — — — — % DCP.

5. The roughages which can not provide maintenance ration when fed alone are called — — — — — — — — — — —.

6. The examples of non-maintenance type roughages are — — — — — — — — — — and — — — — — —which contain — — — — — — percent DCP.

7. Crops grown from April to June are called — — — — — — — — — —.

8. — — — — — — — — and — — — — — — are leguminous crops.

9. — — — — — — — — and — — — — — — non-leguminous crop.

10. Maize is — — — — — — — — — type of fodder.

11. Jowar is — — — — — — and — — — — — — type of fodder.

12. Bajra is — — — — — — — type of fodder.

13. Teosinte (Mak Chari) is an intergenetic cross between — — — — — and — — —.

14. Oat is — — — — — — — type of crop of the rabi season.

15. Berseem fodder contains — — — — — percent CP and — — — — — — — percent TDN on dry matter basis.

16. Most commonly cultivated grasses are — — — — — —, — — — — — — — and — — — —.

17. Tree leaves of — — — — —, — — — — — — and — — — — — — are most commonly used as ruminant feed.

18. — — — — — — — —, — — — — — and — — — are the main tubers used as animal feed.

19. — — — — —, — — — — — — — and — — — — — are the main roots used as animal feed.

20. After extraction of the sugar from sugar beet, the residue is called — — — — —.

21. Two valuable by-products from sugar beet factory are — — — — and — — — —.

22. Roughages contain — — — — percent TDN and — — — — — percent CF.

23. The by-product left after the extraction of oil from oil seeds is called — — — —.

24. Solvent extracted cakes contain — — — — — percent ether extract.

25. The toxic factor present in cotton seed cake is — — — — — — — —.

26. When upper covering of cotton seed is removed to form cake, than — — — — cake is formed.

27. Decorticated cotton seed cake contains — — — — — — crude fibre than under corticated cakes.

28. — — — — — is the toxic factor of linseed cake.

29. Ground nut cake contains the toxic factor known as — — — — — — —.

30. The toxic factor of til seed cake is — — — — — — — — — — —.

31. Mustard seed cake contains — — — — — — — — — — — as a toxic factor.

32. When husks are removed from wheat flour, the product is called — — — — —.

33. — — — — — — — — is a byproduct during process of pulse making.

34. After removal of starch and germ from maize, we obtain — — — — — —.

35. Bone meal is rich source of — — — — — — — — — — and — — — — — — — — — — — — — — — —.

36. Feather meal is rich in protein content and used primarily for feeding of — — — —   — — and — — — — — — — — — — — — — — — — — — —.

37. Linseed meal has a protective action against — — — — — — — — — poisoning.

38. The — — — — — — — — content in potato is higher because it is associated with starch.

39. The main tubers used in livestock feeding are — — — — — — — — — — —, — — — — — — — — — and — — — — — — — — — —.

40. The common antinutritional factors present in tree leaves are — — — — — — — —, — — — — — — — — and — — — — — — — — — — — — — —.

Q.2. Explain the following:

1. Classify the roughages on the basis of nutrient density and season of cultivation.

2. Differentiate between roots and tubers an their impor- tance as animal feed.

3. Importance of grasses and tree leaves in animal nutrition.

4. Define and classify the cakes.

5. Mention the various toxic factors present in different cakes.

6. Tabulate the classification of various feeds and fodder of animal nutrition.

Chapter 2

Conservation of Green Fodder in Animal Nutrition

Feeding of green and succulent fodder is of great importance to farm animals. But the availability of green fodder is limited to a particular season only. During the lean months of May, June, October and November, green fodders are not available for feeding to the livestock. In India, during Kharif season plenty of greens are available but they are not properly utilized by the farmers due to lack of sufficient knowledge of fodder conservation. When conventional feedstuffs are not available to animal for feeding, use of unconventional (i.e. not commonly used for feeding of livestock but used during fodder scarcity period) feeds is being done to maintain the animals and their production. The importance of conservation of fodders is as follows-

● To store surplus fodder during harvesting season.

● To provide good quality fodder during the lean months of the year.

● To maintain the production of animal even during lean period.

So to feed green fodders during lean periods they can be conserved in the form of hay and silage.

Hay making:

Definition of hay: A forage plant when preserved through reducing the moisture content to the level at which plant tissues are dead or dormant is termed as hay.

Advantage of Hay Making:

1. The hay provides the nutritious feed to the livestock during the lean season when there is scarcity of green fodder.

2. The good quality legume hay may reduce the cost of production by replacing certain amount of concentrate in the ration.

3. The fodders can be harvested at the stage when there is maximum accumulation of nutrients in the plant.

4. The ration of the animals can be balanced with the help of good quality hay.

Crops for Hay Making: The legumes crops are preferred for hay making which have soft, thin and pliable stem. Berseem, lucerne, oat, cowpea, soyabean, anjan and sudan grasses are suitable crops for hay making. Some self-grown grasses during mansoon are also used for this purpose.

Method of Hay Making: The fodder or grasses used in hay making processed to reduce the moisture level below 15 percent. The various methods of hay making are described as:

1. Jungle hay: The reserve forests, community forests and pastures are full of perennial grasses and legume mixtures. These are multicut in nature, so, even after several cuttings there is a lot of surplus fodder left behind unharvested in the field till the end of rainy season. The forage mixtures are then harvested and preserved for the feeding of livestock during lean season. These dried out forages are usually termed as jungle hay. Although the method through which the jungle hay is prepared, the forages mixture losses its nutritive value due to low protein and poor digestibility.

2. Sun Drying: The harvested forages can be processed using different ways to reduce the moisture content to a safe. level for preservation. The forage mixtures after harvesting are dried in the field condition with frequent turning of the material. The forages are sometime pooled together to form a poola. These poolas are then kept vertically in the field in the shape of a cone. Sometime the fodder crops after harvesting is spread over in the layer on the barbed wire fencing or boundary wall of the farm or tripod or pyramid which is made of three wooden or iron pieces with an average height 2.5 to 3 meters. It is tilted once or twice before storages for proper curing.

3. Barn drying: The hay can be prepared while storing the forage mixture in a barn. The barn, which is generally used for this purpose have false floor or a system to facilitate the air blowing from ground surface with the help of draft blowers. The air which is blown may be heated or unheated. This type of process is not in practice in the Indian sub-continent.

Advantages of Barn drying:

1. The forages may be baled before drying, thus reducing the cost of transportation to the drying site.
2. The drying time is reduced.
3. The loss of nutrients which occur due to rain is avoided as the process is performed in a barn.
4. The loss of leaves is less to that of field curing.

Disadvantages:

1. The drying is not uniform as the layer facing the blower dries rapidly than that of the opposite layer.
2. The cost of drying is high.
3. The process is not suitable under the high humidity conditions.
4. The turning is not possible for uniform drying.

4. Dehydration of forages: The nutrient loss is high due to handling and plant enzyme activity. The process involves forced hot air ciruclation for rapid drying of the forages. Differed types of drier like low temperature drier, high temperature drier and solar drier are used for dehydration of forages.

Advantages:

1. The forages are dried at a fast rate.
2. The loss due to plant enzyme is minimised.
3. The loss of plant parts mainly leaves is low due to lesser handling during the process.

4. Bales of forage can also be dried.

Disadvantages:

1. High cost involved during establishment and maintenance of dehydration plant.
2. High cost of processing if sufficient amount of forages are not available for dehydration to run the plant continuously.
3. The operation skill is required.

Losses during hay making: The main aim of hay making is to reduce the moisture content of the herbage to a safe level (about 15%) and to retain its nutritional characteristics during the process. Various factors are responsible for the loss of nutritional characteristics of the forage to a variable degree given below.

1. Physical losses: The leaves of forage plants are rich in proteins and also more palatable to the animals than that of the stem usually get separated from the plant during the process of drying. The physical losses are variable depending on the handling and processing of hay making.

2. Chemical losses: The fresh forage plant contains various chemical constituents apart from the water. The loss of water is desirable during the process of hay making while the loss of other components which may reduce nutritional value is undesirable. The losses of chemical constituents which are brought about by plant enzymes, respiration activity and processing method are difficult to measure in field conditions.

1. The enzymes act on soluble carbohydrates and convert them into carbon dioxide and water.
2. The plant proteases start working immediately after the harvesting and are responsible for the loss of nitrogenous fraction.
3. The vitamins A, D and E are mostly affected by drying process. The carotenes, a precursor of vitamin A is unstable in light and air.
4. A considerable loss of carotenes occurs from the action of lipoxidase.

3. Loss of nutritive value: The loss of nutrients is variable in various processes. The chemical constituents of nutritional importance like carbohydrates, nitrogenous substances and vitamins etc. are known to reduce during the process of hay making.

Characteristic of Good hays:

1. It should have a typical aroma of the forage from which it has been prepared. Moisture content should not exceed 15-20 percent.

2. It should be free from foreign material like dust, moulds and undesirable weeds.

3. It should possess reasonable green colour, which gives a rough idea of carotene content.

4. It should maintain leafiness of original fodder. The loss of leaves during the process will produce a poor quality product.

5. It should be palatable to animals. The poorly prepared hay generally is not readily accepted by the animals.

6. Leguminous hay contain 9-15% DCP and 50-60% TDN while gram hay contain contain 2-4% DCP and 45-50% TDN.

Storage of Hay: The forage dried by above methods should contain moisture upto 15 percent. Under drying may result in the development of fermentation and formation of poor quality hay. There is loss of leaves, green colouring matter, and certain nutrient like carbohydrates and vitamins by fermentation, leaching and shattering etc. during the process of storage of hay. These losses can be prevented by storage of hay. The hay is generally stored in the different forms like loose hay, chopped hay, baled hay, and pelleted hay.

Silage making:

Definition of silage: Silage is the green material produced by controlled fermentation of the green fodder crop retaining the high moisture content and maintaining anaerobic conditions, allowing lactobacilli or other similar species to proliferate and produce lactic acid and restricting the growth of spore forming anaerobes and clostridia which produce amines, ammonia and carbondioxide. The process of silage making is called as ensiling. The invention of the baler and plastic wrapping has made it much advantage of the benefits of silage as a supplementary feed for livestock. The high protein green leaf is maintained with only about 20 percent of the nutrients lost in the silage making process. Upto 30 percent of the original nutrients can be lost if silage is made poorly.

Wastelage: It may be defined as a material obtained after ensiling of waste material (animal organic waste) in a suitable combination with forages and additives, under anaerobic conditions, through fermentation by lactic acid producing bacteria.

Advantages of Ensiling:

1. Silage can be prepared from green fodder when the weather does not permit for hay making.

2. Surplus green fodder abundantly available in rainy season can be preserved as silage for feeding during lean season.

3. Silage can be prepared from plants having thick and solid stems that are generally not very suitable for hay making like jowar and maize. Crop should be rich in sugars and starch.

4. Weeds can also be utilized along with main fodder crops for silage making. Silage making destroyed majority of weed seeds.

5. It is highly palatable. Silage from cereal fodder contains about 2-4% DCP and 50-63% TDN.

6. The organic acid produced in the silage are similar to those normally produced in the digestive tract of the ruminants and therefore are used in the same manner.

7. There is lesser loss of carotenes in silage making than that of hay making.

8. Fear of loss due to spontaneous fire sometime experienced in hay making is not there.

9. Green fodder can be stored for a very long period by silage making.

10. The inclusion of raw organic wastes (poultry litter, pig waste etc.) is possible in ruminant diet through ensiling it with forages.

Disadvantages of Ensiling:

1. Transportation of silage is difficult.

2. Permanent structures for preparing silage are required.

3. Wastage during silage making may be high due to affluents losses.

4. Poorly prepared silages are not accepted by animals.

Suitable Crops for Silage Making: The suitable crops for silage making are forages which contain adequate amount of fermentable carbohydrates like maize, jowar, bajra, etc. So non-leguminous crops are more suitable than leguminous crops. However, leguminous fodder can also be used for silage making even they contain less amount of carbohydrates. For that molasses or minerals should be sprinkled over them or mixed with non-leguminous fodder at the time of silage making. The crop for silage making should be harvested at flowering stage as they contain maximum amount of nutrients at that time. The crop should be harvested in the morning after the dew has dried off and should be spread over the field, till noon under the sun rays so that some moisture may be dried up. In the afternoon the crop is collected in bundles.

Silo: The specialized device or containers used for the preparation of silage are called silo. The silos are trench silo, silo tower and silo pit may be rectangular or cylindrical. Based on materials used in construction silo can be made up of brick, cement, stainless steel and kachcha sand. Kachcha silo is prepared by digging a pit or trench in the ground. The sides and floor of silo are generally plastered with a mixture or cow dung and clay (1:1) for making the wall and floor smooth.

Site selection of silo:

1. Site should be easily approachable from field as well as dairy farm.
2. The area should not be low lying, because such type of areas are prone to water logging.
3. The chaffing shed should be adjacent to the site.

Characteristics of Silos: For the preparation of good silage, the silo should have air tight walls without any cracks to avoid entry of rain water which, otherwise spoil the silage. The walls of silo should be smooth and strong without corners. The depth of the silo depends upon the water table in the soil. It should always be above the water table. Similarly, the height of silo will depend upon the machinery available for filling the tower silos. In our country since filling is done by manual labour normally silos are not more than 2-3 m above ground level.

Filling of Silos: Silos can be filled with long fodder as well as with chopped fodder. Chopping is helpful for better packing to minimize the loss of nutrients and chaffed fodder filling and removal of silage is easier.

After chaffing and ensuring that dry matter is around 35 percent the silo is filled with the fodder. The fodder should be evenly distributed throughout the pit. The trampling should be done properly either with men or bullock cart or tractor depending upon the size of pit. At the top, the fodder should be filled in 1.5 m higher than the ground level. From all sides it should be covered with long paddy straw or poor quality grasses and then covered with wet mud and bhusha to seal the materials so that air and water cannot go inside the packed material. The layer of straw/ grasses may be between 4–5 inches. The silage would be prepared in 4-6 weeks after covering.

Process of Ensiling: The process of ensiling begins with the cutting of crops. The respiration activity continues till the silo is closed and acidic conditions are achieved in the silo. The whole process may be divided into four different phases:

Phase I: The phase I immediately start after sealing the tightly filled silo. The plant cells continue to respire till the trapped oxygen is exhausted so length of phase I depends upon the amount of oxygen present in the silo. The carbondioxide produced make the silo anaerobic. Thus, favours the growth of anaerobic bacteria.

Phase II: At the initial stage clostridia and coliform bacteria are active, causing degradation of protein and amino acid and production of amine and acetic acid. Lactic acid producing bacteria are also increased.

Phase III: The lactic acid producing bacteria dominate which increased lactic acid content and reduced pH of ensiled material. The presence of readily available carbohydrate enhanced the growth of such types of desired bacterial population.

Phase IV: This phase is quite variable and dependent on phase III. If pH is reduced to around 4.0 the silage is stable and no further degradation occur. If sufficient acid is not produced to bring down the pH around 4.0 the microbial activity still continues. The degradation of lactic acid to butyric acid starts which spoils the smell and acceptability of silage, through the action of clostridia. High moisture contents favour this undesirable fermentation.

Reaction inside the silo pit (Changes during ensilage): The ensiling is a very complicated process and many changes occur during ensiling. The loss of dry matter, carbohydrate, proteins and pigment occur invariable during fermentation process of silage making. The changes may be biological or chemical in nature and their intensity depend upon the physical and chemical characteristics of ensiled material, compactness of filling and moisture content of ensiled material.

1. Microbiological changes: At initial stage, the aerobic type microbes dominate. The activity of aerobic micro-organisms gradually ceased with the development of anaerobic condition. These are then replaced by fast multiplying anaerobic bacteria such as *Escherchia, Klebsiella, Bacillus, Clostridium, Streptococcus,*

Leuconostoc, Lactobacillus and *Pediococcus*. Being facultative anaerobes, yeasts present in the silo contents also proliferate in the silage. Growth of micro-organism in ensiling materials are influenced by moisture content of forages, soluble carbohydrates, mechanical processes and additives added to the ensiled materials.

2. Chemical changes in ensiling:

Changes in carbohydrates: Monosaccharides (glucose and fructose) and disaccharides (sucrose) are the dominating water soluble carbohydrates in forages. Oligosaccharides other than sucrose are present in low quantity. The components which are utilized maximum during the processof ensiling are the soluble carbohydrates as polysaccharide and oligosaccharides present in green forage which are hydrolyzed as-

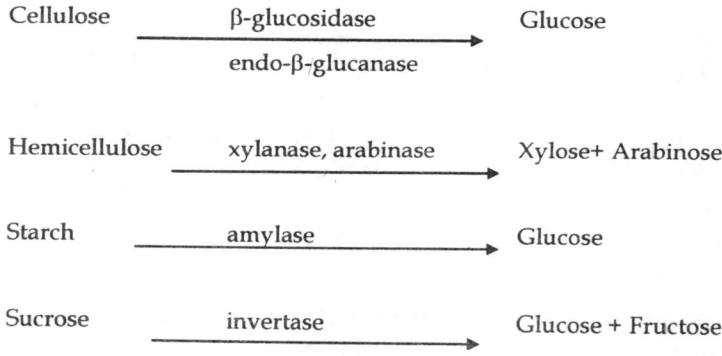

Cellulose	β-glucosidase / endo-β-glucanase	→	Glucose
Hemicellulose	xylanase, arabinase	→	Xylose+ Arabinose
Starch	amylase	→	Glucose
Sucrose	invertase	→	Glucose + Fructose

The chemical changes take place by plant enzyme in initial stage then microbial fermentation take place.

(a) Plant enzymes: The plant cells remains active and respire till the oxygen of silo is lost. They utilize soluble carbohydrates and convert them into carbondioxide and water.

$$C_6H_{12}O_6 + 6 O_2 \longrightarrow 6 H_2O + 6 CO_2 + 673 \text{ K cal}$$

(b) Microbial degradation of carbohydrate: The carbohydrates glucose, fructose, xylose and arabinose, are degraded by lactic acid producing bacteria. The degradation of various carbohydrates take place by homo lactic and heterolactic fermentation and produce various fermentative products such as lactic acid, acetic acid, mannitol and carbondioxide. The number of lactic acid producing bacteria is usually low in fresh forage and most of these bacteria are heterofermentative. Heterofermentative lactic acid bacteria produce less organic acid than homofermentative and some of energy is lost in the form of carbon dioxide which is responsible for the loss of energy of the forages during the ensiling process. This loss can be minimized by using a inoculum of a homofermentative lactic acid producing bacteria in the premix before filling in the silo.

The degradation products of homo lactic and heterolactic fermentation of hexoses and pentoses are given below:

S.No.	Substrate	Type of fermentation	End products.
1.	Glucose + ADP (1 mole)	Homolactic fermentation	Lactic acid + 2 ATP (2 mole)
2.	Fructose + 2 ADP (2 mole)	Homolactic fermentation	Lactic acid + 2 ATP (2 mole)
3.	Glucose + ADP (1 mole)	Homolactic fermentation	Lactic acid + Ethanol + CO_2 + ATP (1 mole)
4.	Fructose + 2 ADP + H_2O (3 mole)	Heterolactic fermentation	Lactic acid (1 mole) + Mannitol (2 mole) +Acetic acid (1 mole) + CO_2 + 2 ATP
5.	Arabinose + 2 ADP (1 mole)	Homo and heterolactic fermentation	Lactic acid (1 mole) + Acetic acid (1 mole) + 2 ATP
6.	Xylose + 2 ADP (1 mole)	Homo and heterolactic fermentation	Lactic acid (1 mole) + Acetic acid (1 mole) + 2 ATP

Microbial degradation of organic acids: Forages generally contain proportionally higher quantities of citric acid and malic acid, which are degraded both by homo and heterolactic bacteria. Degradation products of organic acid by homo and heterolactic fermentation are lactic acid, acetic acid, formic acid, ethanol and 2, 3 butanediol.

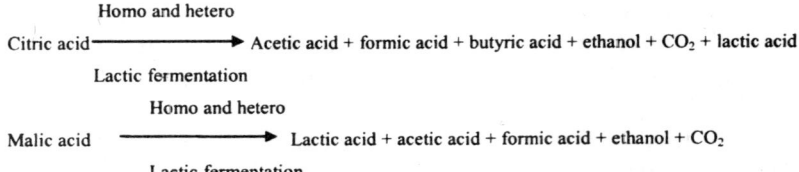

Homo and hetero

Citric acid ⟶ Acetic acid + formic acid + butyric acid + ethanol + CO_2 + lactic acid

Lactic fermentation

Homo and hetero

Malic acid ⟶ Lactic acid + acetic acid + formic acid + ethanol + CO_2

Lactic fermentation

Chemical changes in nitrogenous compound:

The degradation of nitrogenous compounds during ensiling is caused by plant enzymes and microbes of aerobic or anaerobic nature.

1. Plant enzymes: The changes in the nitrogenous fraction and degradation of protein to non-protein nitrogen (NPN) is carried out by plant enzymes. The activity of plant enzyme is dependent on moisture content of forage and pH of ensiled material. The plant proteolytic activity is high during high moisture level in forages. The leaf proteases are more active in a pH range of 5.0 to 6.0. Apart from the hydrolysis of proteins further breakdown of amino acid is also possible. Below pH 4.3, the proteolytic activity of plant enzymes is ceased. A slow rate of wilting associated with slow decline in pH may cause extensive loss of proteinous fractions of ensiled forages by proteolytic activity.

2. Microbial degradation of nitrogenous compound: Proteins are broken down into amino acids by microbial degradation in well preserved silage. There are many different types of microbes like lactobacilli, pediococcus, sterptococcus and clostridium etc. which are present in the content of silo. The degradation of nitrogenous source is variable depending on the nature of bacteria, rate of pH decline and nature of crops etc.

In badly preserved silage the amino acid are further broken down to produce various amines like tryptamine, phenyl-ethlamine and histamine. The principal products of putrification are betaine, adenine and pentamethylene diamine.

Pigments: The colour of the forages usually changes on

ensiling. The light brown colour or golden yellow colour is caused by the action of organic acid on chlorophyll. The phacophytin is the resultant of this reaction.

Flavour and aroma: A well prepared silage with lactic acid fermentation has its characteristics flavour and aroma. It has been observed that even off flavour and aroma of pig waste can be converted to pleasant fruity smell after ensiling with forage and molasses.

Losses during ensilage: The losses of nutrient during ensiling include all type of losses arising from processes involved from harvesting of forage in the field to finishing product (silage). These losses which occur during the process of silage are discussed below:

1.   **Field losses:** The losses occur after the harvesting of crop till it is filled in the silo are considered field losses. These losses may be due to shattering of leaves and other nutritious plant parts after harvesting the forage. Apart from the handling, the loss of dry matter may be due to tissue respiration and activity of plant enzymes during the process of wilting.

2.   **Aerobic fermentation:** During the process of filling the silo pit, the air pocket, are usually left in side pit. The air present in silo causing aerobic fermentation of carbohydrates. The extent of losses due to aerobic fermentation processes is directly and positively related with the amount of air present in the silo.

3.   **Anaerobic fermentation losses:** The losses of dry matter due to anaerobic fermentation processes may be of water soluble carbohydrates, proteins, and organic acids. The intensity however, depends on the nature of microorganism dominating of forage and the rate of decline in pH. The losses of dry matter due to anaerobic fermentation may range to 2-10 percent of heavily wilted forage samples.

4.   **Effluent losses:** As effluent production in the silo is responsible for a considerable loss of nutrients, when forage of high moisture content (more than 70 percent) is ensiled. The

loss of dry matter recorded upto 10-80 percent when formic acid used as a preservative for lush green forage. The effluent production is influenced by following factors:

(a) Moisture content of ensiled forage

(b) Degree of compactness

(c) Pre-treatment of ensiled forage

(d) Preservative used

(e) Nature of crops

(f) Fermentation processes

The effluent production is directly and positively related with the moisture content of forages. This correlation is true with the forages having more than 70 percent moisture. In the forage with less than 70 percent moisture level the effluent production is negligible. The legumes are mostly harvested at succulent stage, so care should be taken to avoid the loss due to effluent production through mixing it either with dry fodder or low moisture forages.

Procedure for preparation of good silage: To get a good silage one should take care at every stage of ensiling. A few precautions required to be taken are given below:

1. **Harvesting of crop:** The ensiling does not add nutrients to the forage but it preserves the nutrients of the herbage. The necessary precaution should be taken to select a suitable stage of forage for harvesting maximum nutrients. The boot of half bloom stage is suitable in single cut forage while multicut crops can be harvested at 55-60 days after sowing for first cut and after 25-30 days for subsequent cuttings.

2. **Wilting of crop to 30-40 percent dry matter:** The loss of dry matter is more due to effluent production which is associated with high moisture content of ensiled material, so the wilting of crop to reduce moisture content to 60-65 per cent is desirable.

3. **Chaffing of forages:** Chaffed forages can be compressed to a greater extent and it exposes more plant surface area for faster microbial growth and lactic acid production.

4. **Mixing of legume and non-legume crops**: The legumes are rich sources of protein with low level of carbohydrates whereas non-legumes are poor in protein and rich sources of carbohydrates. When both are mixed together, they can be turned into good quality silage.

5. **Mixing of additives**: There are many types of additives being used in ensilage. These may be stimulators or inhibitors of microbial activities in silage. These are a follows:

   (a) Inorganic chemicals. Calcium carbonate, magnesium carbonate, ammonium sulphate, sodium sulphate, zinc sulphate, copper sulphate, ferrous sulphate, manganese sulphate, sodium chloride, sodium nitrites, calcium phosphate, calcium silicate and phosphoric acid.

   (b) Organic chemicals. Acetic acid, citric acid, benzoic acid, formic acid, lactic acid, propionic acid, formaldehyde, ethyl alcohol, propylene glycol, lactate, sodium gluconate, ethyl acetate, ethyl butyrate, ethyl diamine dihydro iodide and urea etc.

   (c) Feed stuffs. Used as silage additives are wheat bran, crushed maize, starch, dextrose, molasses, whey and ·yeast etc.

   (d) Fermentation products and micro-organisms. A few enzymes like malt diastase and extract of fungi and several species of micro-organisms like lactobacilus acidophilus, torulopsis sp., Bacillus subtilis etc. have been used for enhanced silage production.

6. **Filling of silo**: The well compressed packing of silage will help the creation of anaerobic condition earliest causing the production of good silage.

7. **Sealing of silo**: The air-tight sealing is necessary to avoid the entrance of air in the silo.

8. **Removal of silage**: After a period of 4-6 weeks the silage is ready for feeding to the livestock. After the removal of silage, the open end of the silo should be covered in such a manner that the contact from the air is minimum.

Special Methods of Silage Making: Excellent silage can be produced from legumes and other grasses when ground grain or other concentrates are added to the green fodder. This is a practice in U.S.A. It is not at all practised in our country.

A.I.V. method: This method is named after the name of its originator A.I. Virtanen. In the A.I.V. method, a mixture of sulphuric acid and hydrochloric acid is added to the forage to bring the pH below 4.0. The resultant mixture is preserved for a sufficiently long period. Cattle are able to consume the silage without any detrimental effect. This method of silage making is not at all practised in our country..

Artificial drying of grasses: In some agriculturally advanced countries leguminous forage are dehydrated. The forage is first chaffed and is passed through the drier, where it is exposed to hot air. Dehydration preserve the nutritive value of the fodders better than the field cured hay but it is very costly and is not at all practised in our country on commercial scale. Artificially dried berseem, Lucerne etc. can be used as a protein supplement in pigs and poultry rations also.

Extraction of leaf protein concentrates: The proteins are present in the cell content of the forages. The whole processes involve following steps and the quantity and quality of leaf protein concentrates depends on the processing.

1. **Selection of crops:** Succulent and juicy forage with high levels of protein is usually preferred for the extraction of leaf protein. The legumes like berseem, lucerne and cowpea etc. can be good source of leaf protein. Immature young crops of wheat and oats are also harvested for the extraction of leaf protein concentrates.

2. **Harvesting of crops:** The protein and water contents of plants diminish with the increasing age of plant. Protein and water content are the main responsible factors affecting the yield of the leaf proteins. With the maturity the carbohydrates content of the cell wall increases which adversely affect the extraction of plant proteins. The early harvesting is, therefore, required for extract the maximum cell content.

3. **Extraction of crop:** The juice from the forages may be extracted by different methods depending upon the several factors like extracting efficiency of the method, capacity of the extraction, type of the crop etc. commonly used sugarcane juice extractors may be used for this purpose.

4. **Processing of juice:** The juice extracted from plants contains many chemical constituents other than proteins. Separation of protein from other undesirable plant constituents involves many steps and the quality of plant protein is affected by the processing steps. Various types of leaf protein concentrates has been developed for human consumption but their acceptability is poor because due to slightly bitter taste, strong grassy flavour and green colour. This can be easily used in the diet of pigs, poultry and other animals replacing costlier and scarce sources of conventional proteins. The cost of leaf protein preparation for the feeding of animals can be reduced by eliminating a few steps of processing like removal of colour and smell etc.

Haylage: It is a low moisture silage (40-45% moisture) made from grass or legume that is wilted to 40-45 percent moisture content before ensiling.

Q.1. Fill in the blanks.

1. Green fodders are conserved by the process of — — — — and — — — —.
2. Best crop for hay making is — — — — — — — —.
3. The hay to be stored should contain — — — — — percent moisture.
4. The suitable crops for hay making should be harvested at — — — — — stage.
5. The vitamins — — — — — — and — — — — — — are most affected by drying process during hay making.
6. The best hay should contain — — — — percent dry matter.
7. There is less loss of — — — — — — — in silage making than that of hay making.
8. The best crop for silage making is — — — — — — — — —.

9. The container used for silage making is — — — — — — —.
10. For silage making the dry matter content of crop should be — — — — — percent.
11. — — — — — — — — —, — — — — — — and — — — — — — — are the anaerobic microbes which proliferate in the silage.
12. The pH value of good silage is — — — — — — —.
13. The soluble carbohydrates are degraded into — — — — and — — — — — — —.
14. — — — — — — — — — and — — — — — — type of fermentation will take place during microbial degradation of carbohydrates in silage making.
15. A good silage has — — — — odour and — — — — — — — — — colour.
16. On fermentation, glucose breaks down into — — — — — — and — — — — — — — — —.
17. Growth of the microorganisms in ensiling materials is influenced by — — — — — — and — — — — — — — — — — — — — — — — — —.
18. Green fodder can be stored for a longer period by — — — — — — — — — — making.
19. Kachcha silo is prepared by — — — — — — — — — — — — — — — — — in the ground.

Q.2. Explain the following.
1. Advantage of hay making.
2. Losses occur during the process of hay making.
3. Define the term "hay". What are the suitable crops for hay making?
4. Characteristics of good silage.
5. What are the advantages of silage making over hay making?
6. What is a silo? Explain the type of silo and characteristics of silo.
7. Explain the various process of ensiling.
8. Explain the changes occur during ensiling.
9. What are the losses occur during ensiling?
10. Explain the procedure for preparation of good silage.

Chapter 3

Evaluation of Energy Value of Feed in Animal Nutrition

Definition of energy: Energy is defined as the capacity to do work. As we know, heat is measured in some units known as calories which may be defined as follows:

1. **Calorie (Cal):** The amount of energy as heat required to raise the temperature of 1 gram of water to 1 °C (precisely from 14.5°C to 15.5°C). One cal is equal to 4.184 Joule.

2. **Kilocalorie (K cal):** The amount of energy as heat required to raise the temperature of 1 kg of water to 1°C (from 14.5°C to 15.5°C). Kilocalorie is equivalent to 1000 calories.

3. **Megacaloria (M cal):** Equivalent to 1000 kilocalories or 1000,000 calories, formerly referred to as a therm.

4. **British thermal unit (BTU):** The amount of energy as heat required to raise the temperature of 1 pound of water to 1°F. It is equal to 252 calories.

5. **Joule (J):** The International Union of Nutritional Sciences and the nomenclature committee of the International Union of Physiological Sciences have suggested the Joule (J) as the unit of energy for use in nutritional, metabolism and physiological studies.

The Joule is defined as 1 newton metre, and 1 J = 0.24 cal. kilo joule (KJ) and mega joule (MJ), are also explained similarly.

The simplest method for measuring the value of any feed is to determine the amount of digestible nutrients that is supplied to the animals. For expressing the energy value of feeds and requirements of animals, following systems are used.

1. Total digestible nutrients (TDN)
2. Starch equivalent (SE)
3. Gross energy (GE)
4. Digestible energy (DE)
5. Metabolizable energy (ME)
6. Net energy (NE)
7. Scandinavian feed unit.

1. Total digestible nutrients (TDN): TDN is simply a figure which indicates the relative energy value of a feed to an animal. It is ordinarily expressed in pounds or kilogram's or in percent (pound or kg of TDN per 100 pound or kg of feed). It is arrived at by adding together the following:

TDN percent = Percent digestible crude protein + Percent digestible crude fibre + Percent digestible nitrogen- free extract + Percent digestible ether extract × 2.25

% TDN = % DCP + % DCF + % DNFE + % DEE × 2.25.

Fat on oxidation provides 2.25 time more energy as compared to carbohydrates, hence the figure is multiple by 2.25. The protein in this equation has been included because of the fact that excess of protein eaten by the animals serve as a source of energy to the body.

Limitation of the TDN System:
1. It over estimates the value of roughages because more energy spent in chewing of such feeds remains unaccounted.
2. Only the loss in faeces is accounted.
3. If feeds are high in fat content will some time exceed 100 in percentage of TDN.

Factors affecting the TDN value of a feed:

1. The percentage of the dry matter. The more water present in feed, the less there is of other nutrients, and lowers the TDN value.

2. **The digestibility of the dry matter.** Unless the dry matter of a feed is digestible, it can have no TDN value. Only digestible dry matter can contribute TDN. Lignin has a high energy value but it can not be digested by the animals so has no digestible energy or TDN values.

3. **The amount of mineral matter in the digestible dry matter.** Mineral contribute no energy to the animal though mineral compounds are digestible but have no TDN value. The more mineral matter a feed contains, other things being equals, the lower will be its TDN values.

4. **The amount of fat in the digestible dry matter.** Fat contributes 2.25 times as much as energy per unit of weight as do carbohydrates and protein. The feeds high in digestible fat some time TDN value exceed 100%. In fact, a pure fat which had a coefficient of digestibility of 100 percent would theoretically have a TDN value of 225% (100 × 2.25 = 225).

Thus we find that the digestibility data obtained from the simple digestion trial is of a very limited application, but the animals shall have to feed on the basis of some standard. The Morrison feeding standard is based on the total digestible nutrients, obtained from carefully conducted digestion trials.

2. The starch equivalent: Kellner, measured the values of feeds for productive purposes in terms of strach values, instead of net energy values stated in therms. In this system 1 pound of digestible starch is taken as the net energy unit. Suppose the starch equivalent of wheat bran is 45 kg it means that 100 kg of the wheat bran can produce as much animal fat as 45 kg of pure starch when fed in addition to maintenance ration or in other words 100 kg of wheat bran contain as much net or productive energy as 45 kg of the starch. The starch equivalent can be calculated as:

$$SE = \frac{\text{Weight of fat stored per unit of food}}{\text{Weight of fat stored per unit weight of starch}} \times 100$$

Kellner added pure carbohydrate, protein and fat to a basal maintenance ration to determine the relative amounts of these pure digestible nutrients required to produce a unit of body fat using the nitrogen-carbon balance method.

One kg of digestible proteins produces 235 grams of fat

One kg of digestible starch and cellulose produces 248 grams of fat.

One kg of digestible cane sugar produces 188 grams of fat.

One kg of digestible fat produces 474 to 598 grams of fat.

Taking starch as the unit, the fat producing power of protein, fat and carbohydrate was then calculated as follows:

One part digestible protein $= \dfrac{235}{248} = 0.95$ (SE)

One part of digestible fat $= \dfrac{474}{248}$ to $\dfrac{598}{248} 1.91$ to 2.41 (SE)

One part of digestible starch $= \dfrac{248}{248} = 1.00$ (SE)

Kellner conceived that the ether extract from oil cake (which is more or less pure oil) and the same extract from a green plant could not have the equal fat producing capacity or SE value and suggested the following multiplication factors to be used in the calculation of SE.

	Factor
One part of digestible fat from coarse fodders like green or dry roughage (straws, hays, silage and green grasses)	1.91
One part of digestible fat from brans and other grains or grain products	2.12
One part of digestible fat from oilseed, oilcakes and other animal products	2.41

100 grams feed (On dry matter basis)	Body fat in calories	
	Calculated value	Observed values
Cotton seed meal	191.40	186.90
Linseed cake	186.80	182.80
Palm-kernel	170.50	173.90
Groundnut meal	179.50	179.80
Wheat straw	98.90	20.10
Oat straw	103.60	62.80
Barley straw	111.10	74.70
Meadow hay	122.80	77.10
Clover hay	118.30	81.10

Kellner also compared the observed and calculated value. The observed and the calculated values agreed remarkably well in cakes and meals but differ with coarse feed stuffs like straws and hays. He realized that there should be some difference between the efficiency of utilization of a straw and oil cakes. The descripancy was explained on the basis of the crude fibre content of the feeds. Kellner conceived that more fibrous was the food, the greater was the expenditure of energy in chewing, mastication, digestion etc. In fact he demonstrate that if the fodder was chopped and fed, for every gram of crude fibre eaten, the expenditure of energy was 0.70 calorie, whereas, when fed unchopped, energy spent was 1.36 calories for the same fodder. This means that chopping itself reduces the expenditure of energy by half. He finally suggested the use of the following factors for the calculation of starch equivalent.

Type of fodder	Percentage of crude fibre to be multiplied by the factor
1. Dry roughages (Straw, hay etc.)	0.58
2. Dry roughages finely chopped	0.29
3. Green fodder (Percentage of fibre on wet basis)	
4.0	0.29
5.0	0.31
6.0	0.34
7.0	0.36

8.0	0.38
9.0	0.40
10.0	0.43
11.0	0.45
12.0	0.48
13.0	0.50
14.0	0.53
15.0	0.55
16.0 or more	0.58

It was observed that when dry straw such as wheat or paddy are chopped, the expenditure of energy in chewing and mastication is almost similar to that of a green roughage containing only 4 per cent of crude fibre.

Examples for the calculation of SE:

1. Concentrates such as linseed cake:

Nutrients	% digestible nutrients	Factor	SE
Crude protein	24.0	0.95	22.80
Ether extract	9.0	2.40	21.60
Nitrogen-free extract	29.0	1.00	29.00
Crude fibre	5.0	1.00	5.00
		Total	78.50

In case of concentrates like oilseed cake, no deduction for fibre is needed. The digestible nutrients are only multiplied by a value number. Such value number mostly range between 95 and 100 in the case of oil cakes. The value number of linseed cake is 97.0. Therefore, the SE value is 78.40 × 0.97 kg per 100 kg of materials.

2. Green fodder such as berseem:

Nutrients	% digestible Nutrients	Factor	SE
Crude protein	2.0	0.95	1.90
Ether extract	0.5	1.91	1.00
Total carbohydrates	9.0	1.00	9.00
		Total	11.90
Content of crude fibre on wet basis = 6.0 %			11.90
Therefore, deduct 6 × 0.34 = 2.04			- 2.04
			9.86

Hence 100 kg of green berseem contain 9.86 kg of SE. It indicates that SE of green fodder is much less than oil cake.

3. Dry roughage such as hay :

Nutrients	% digestible Nutrients	Factor	SE
Crude protein	4.0	0.95	3.80
Ether extract	1.0	1.91	1.90
Crude fibre	28.0	1.00	28.00
Nitrogen-free extract	13.0	1.00	13.00
Total SE calculated			46.70
Deduct crude fibre 28.0 × 0.58 = 16.20			16.20
		Corrected SE	30.50
Total calculated SE			46.70
Deduct crude fibre 28.0 × 0.29 if the hay is chopped			8.10
		Corrected SE	38.60

Therefore, 100 kg of the hay contains 30.5 kg SE and 38.6 kg SE (if the hay is chopped).

3. Gross energy: Gross energy is the total heat of combustion of a material as determined with a bomb calorimeter and expressed as megajoule/kg dry matter. Some typical gross energy values are shown in table. The gross energy value of a feed has no relationship to the feeds digestible, metabolizable or net energy values, except that the latter can never exceeded the GE. Certain products such as coal, mineral oil and lignin have high gross energy values but, because of their indigestibility have no energy value to the animal. Roughages have high gross energy values comparable to those of concentrates, but the two differ greatly in digestible, metabolizable and net energy values.

Constituents		Gross energy values MJ/Kg DM
1. Food constituents	Glucose	15.60
	Strach	17.70
	Cellulose	17.50
	Casein	24.50
	Butter fat	38.50
	Fat (from oil seeds)	39.00
2. Fermentation products		
	Acetic acid	14.60
	Propionic acid	20.80
	Butyric acid	24.90
	Methane	55.00
3. Animal tissue	Muscle	23.60
	Fat	39.30
4. Feeds	Maize	18.50
	Oat grain	19.60
	Oat straw	18.50
	Linseed oil meal	21.40
	Grass hay	18.90
	Milk (4% Fat)	24.90

4. Digestible energy (DE): This is that portion of the gross energy of a feed which does not appear in the faeces. It includes metabolizable energy as well as the energy of the urine and methane. Considerable quantity of heat of the digested food is eliminated in the faeces. The apparent digestible energy of the food is the gross energy of the feed less the energy contained in faeces.

5. Metabolizable energy (ME): It is that portion of gross energy not appearing in the faeces, urine and gases of fermentation (Principally methane). It is digestible energy minus the energy of the urine and methane. It is comparable to the energy of TDN minus the energy of the fermentation gases.

Metabolizable energy = Gross energy - (energy lost in faeces + energy lost in combustible gases + energy lost in urine).

Normally about 8 percent of the gross energy intake is lost through the methane production. Metabolizable energy can also be calculated from the digestible energy by multiplying with 0.82 which means that about 18 percent of the energy is lost through urine and methane. In poultry, metabolizable energy is measured more easily than digestible energy because the faeces and urine are voided together.

Swift and coworkers gave the following equation for calculation of methane production.

Methane production in sheep = E = 2.41 X + 9.80

Methane production in cattle = E = 4.012 X + 17.68

Where,   E = methane in gram

X = digestible carbohydrates in 100 grams

Methane contains 13.34 k cal of energy per gram.

Factors affecting the Metabolizable Energy values of foods:

1. **Species of animals:** The metabolizable energy of feeding stuffs varies according to the species to which it is being fed. In the ruminants about 8-10 per cent losses of energy are in the methane production while in the non-ruminants there are no such losses. Therefore, the ME values are higher in non-ruminants than ruminants. This gap is more in the feeding stuffs rich in the crude fibre.

2. **Composition of feed:** Chemical composition of the feed also affect the ME values of food. If the crude protein present in the food is unbalanced then the majority of the amino acids will be deaminated and greater proportion of nitrogen will be excreted as urea. One gram of urea excreted will be equivalent to 23.00 KJ of energy. Therefore, generally the ME values are frequently corrected to zero nitrogen balance. For ruminant a factor of 31.17 KJ per gram of nitrogen has been used; for poultry the factor is 34.39 KJ per gram. The crude fibre level also affect the ME value of feed.

3. **Processing of food:** Processing of food also affect the ME values since it affects the losses of nutrients in faeces and methane production.

4. **Level of feeding:** The level at which feed is being fed affect the ME value of the feed. At high level of feed intake ME values are reduced.

6. **Net energy (NE):** This is that portion of metabolizable energy which may be used by the animals for work, growth, fattening, foetal development, milk production, and/or heat production. It differs from metabolizable energy that net energy does not include the heat of fermentation and nutrient metabolism or the heat increment. The fate of the gross energy of food is summarised as:

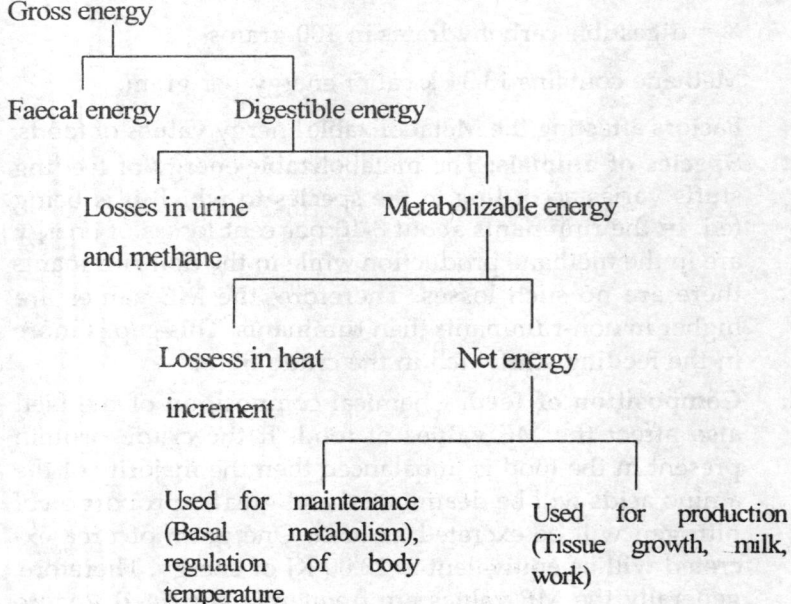

Heat increment of metabolizable energy and net energy used in maintenance is summarized as total heat production of the animal. The heat increment is also known as specific dynamic effect of food. This heat is useful only for keeping an animal warm during very cold weather. At other times the energy represented by this heat is not only a complete loss but also may actually interfere with production by causing the animals to be too warm.

7. Scandinavian feed unit system: In this system one pound of barley grain is taken as the standard. The feed unit value for any other feed is the amount of that feed which is estimated to have the same productive value as 1.00 pound of barley. For example, the feed unit values of soybean oil meal for dairy cows are 0.85 pound and the value for corn grain is 0.95 pound. This means 0.85 1b. of soybean oil meal or 0.95 1b of corn is equal to 1 lbs of barley in feeding value. In this system feeds that are rated below barley in value per pound are given higher numerical values than 1.0. The feed unit value of wheat bran is given 1.25 1bs. This means that it will take 1.25 1bs of wheat bran to equal 1 1bs of barley in value for dairy cows. This system has the merit of comparing the values of feed on the basis of actual result when applied in practice. Consequently any specific value that the feed may possess in addition to its protein and energy values receives proper recognition.

Methods for measuring the heat production and energy retention: There are two ways by which heat production can be measured for determining the net energy values of the feeding stuffs.

1. **Direct calorimetry:** In which heat production is measured directly; this combines the feature of both respiration chamber and calorimeter.

2. **Indirect calorimetry:** In this method net energy is determined by indirect means where only exchange of gases is recorded that means only respiration chamber is needed.

Direct calorimetry: This apparatus was used by Atwater in 1892 for the human beings. After that Armsby built an apparatus for energy metabolism studies for the farm animals. In this apparatus there is a provision for recording the intake of feed, water and oxygen and the outgo of faeces, urine, gaseous excretion and heat loss from the body. The heat is lost from the body through conduction, radiation, convection and evaporation of water from skin and expired gases through lungs.

The animal calorimeter is basically an air tight and insulated chamber. Evaporative losses of heat are measured by recording the volume of air drawn through the chamber and its moisture content on entry and exit are used for calculation of heat loss.

The heat loss through conduction, radiation and convection of the animal is measured by the rise in temperature of the cold water flowing in various pipes suspended in the chamber from ceiling. The rate of flow of water and differences in the temperature at the entry and exist are used for the calculation of heat loss.

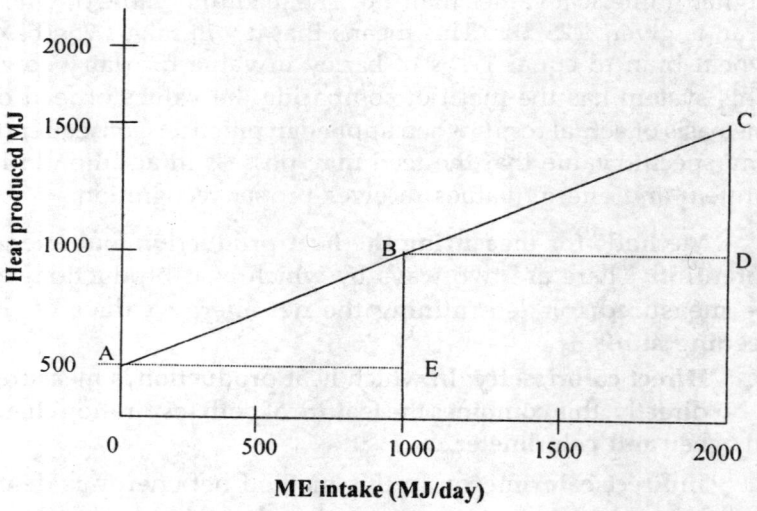

Determination of heat increment:

The heat increment of the feed is determined by feeding two levels of feed intake. The difference in the two levels would give the heat production due to the increase in feed intake. In this case assumption is made that heat production due to basal metabolism would remain the same at both the levels. The increase in heat production at higher intake is due to the additional feed given to the animal. In given example a particular feed was fed to an animal in respiration calorimeter at two levels of metabolizable energy namely 1000 and 2000 MJ. There was an increase in heat production 500 MJ. The heat increment with an increase of 1000 MJ of ME would be:

$$\frac{CD}{BD} \times 100 = \frac{500}{1000} \times 100 = 50 \text{ percent}$$

A is the basal metabolism and B and C represent heat production at metabolizable energy intakes of 1000 and 2000 MJ, respectively. For the sake of simplicity the relation between heat production and metabolizable energy intake is shown here as being linear, i.e. ABC is a straight line.

Animal calorimeters are expensive to build and the earlier types required much labour to operate them. Because of this most animal calorimetry today is carried out by the indirect methods.

Indirect calorimetry: Measurement of heat production by direct calorimetry is costly so, most of the measurements for heat production, are done by indirect method. The heat loss in indirect calorimetry is measured by carbon-nitrogen balance or through gaseous exchange method.

1. Carbon-nitrogen balance method. Carbon and nitrogen enter the body only in the food. Carbon leaves the body through faeces, urine, methane and carbon dioxide and nitrogen leaves the body through faeces and urine only. Therefore, the balance trial must be carried out in a respiration chamber. The procedure for calculating energy retention and heat loss from carbon nitrogen balance data is illustrated by considering an animal in which storage of both fat and protein is taking place. In such an animal intakes of carbon and nitrogen will be greater than the quantity excreted and the animal is said to be a positive balance with respect of these elements. The quantity of protein stored is calculated by multiplying the nitrogen balance by factor 6.25. Protein also contains 51.2 percent (g C/100 g), and the amount of carbon stored as protein can therefore, be computed. The remaining carbon is stored as fat, which contains 74.6 percent.

229

Fat storage is therefore, calculated by dividing the carbon balance, less that stored as protein by 0.746. The energy present in the protein and fat stored is then calculated by using average calorific values for body tissue. These values for cattle and sheep are 3.93 MJ/100 g for fat and 2.36 MJ/100 g of protein. Calculation of the energy retention and heat production of a sheep from carbon nitrogen balance is given below as.

Nutrient	Carbon (g)	Nitrogen (g)	Energy (MJ)
Intake	684.5	41.67	28.41
Excretion in faeces	279.3	13.96	11.47
Excretion in urine	33.6	25.41	1.50
Excretion as methane	20.3	-	1.49
Excretion as carbon dioxide	278.0	-	-
Balance	73.3	2.30	
Intake of metabolizable energy	-	-	13.95
Protein and fat storage			
Protein stored	(2.30 × 6.25)		14.4g
Carbon stored as protein	(14.4 × 0.512)		7.4g
Carbon stored as fat	(73.3 – 7.4)		65.9g
Fat stored	(65.9 ÷ 0.746)		88.3g
Energy retention and heat production			
Energy stored as protein	(14.4 × 23.6)		0.34MJ
Energy stored as fat	(88.3 × 39.3)		3.47MJ
Total energy retention	(0.34 + 3.47)		3.81MJ
Heat production	(13.95 – 3.81)		10.14MJ

Calculation of energy retention and heat production by carbon-nitrogen balance in sheep:

2. **Respiratory exchange of gases method:** These methods take into account the oxygen consumption, carbon dioxide production and urinary nitrogen to calculate the non-protein RQ.

The respiratory quotient (RQ) is the ratio between the volume of carbon dioxide produced and the volume of oxygen used by the animals.

$$RQ = \frac{\text{Volume of carbon dioxide produced}}{\text{Volume of oxygen used}}$$

When carbohydrates are being oxidised in the body for energy purposes the R.Q. is 1 and has been shown by the following equation:

$$C_6H_{12}O_6 + 6\ CO_2 \longrightarrow 6\ CO_2 + 6\ H_2O + 2.82\ MJ.$$

When fats (tripalmitin) are being oxidised in the body for energy purposes the R.Q. is 0.7 and has been shown by following equation:

$$C_3H_5(C_{15}H_{31}COO)_3 + 72.5\ O_2 \longrightarrow 51\ CO_2 + 49\ H_2O + 32.04MJ.$$

The heat of combustion of protein varies according to the amino acid proportion but averages 22.2 KJ/g proteins. The quantity of protein catabolized can be estimated from the output of nitrogen in the urine, 0.16 g of urinary nitrogen being excreted for each gram of protein. For each gram of protein oxidised, 0.77 litre of carbon dioxide is produced and 0.96 litre of oxygen used, giving an RQ of 0.8. In an experiment the following results were obtained:

Oxygen consumed   392.0 litres

Carbon dioxide produced   310.7 litres

Nitrogen excreted in urine   14.8 g

Heat from protein metabolism

Protein oxidised   (14.8 × 6.25) = 92.5g

Heat produced   (92.5 × 18.0) = 1665 KJ

Oxygen used   (92.5 × 0.96) = 88.8 litre

Carbon dioxide   (92.5 × 0.77) = 71.2 litre

Heat from fat and carbohydrate metabolism

Oxygen used   (392.0 – 88.8) = 303.2 litre

Carbon dioxide produced   (310.7 – 71.2) = 239.5 litre

Non-protein RQ   0.79

Thermal equivalent of oxygen when RQ is 0.79 = 20.00 KJ/litre

Heat produced (303.2 × 20.0) = 6064 KJ

Total heat produced (1665 + 6064) = 7729 KJ

For measuring the respiratory exchange in the farm animals two types of respiration chambers have been used.

1. Open circuit respiration chamber,
2. Close circuit respiration chamber.

In both the cases the chamber is air-tight where there is an arrangement for feeding, watering, and milking of the animals. There is arrangement for collection of faeces and urine also.

Brouwer equation: This equation is used for calculation of heat production (H.P.) in Kilojoule.

$$H.P = 16.18\ VO_2 + 5.16\ VCO_2 - 5.90\ N - 2.42\ CH_4$$

Where

VO_2 = Oxygen consumed (litres)

VCO_2 = Carbon dioxide produced (litres)

N = Urinary nitrogen excreted (gram)

CH_4 = Methane production (litres)

For Poultry, the N-coefficient is 1.20 (instead of 5.90) as poultry excrete nitrogen in the more oxidized form of uric acid rather than as urea.

Physiological Fuel Values of Atwater: In human nutrition, Atwater calculated the calorific values of the nutrients which were available for transformation in the body. The following digestibility figures were taken for the nutrients.

Carbohydrates 98%

Fats 95%

Proteins 92%

The calorific values of the nutrient were then multiplied by these coefficients to get the physiological fuel values. In the case of protein 5.23 MJ is substrated per g of protein in order to account for the energy lost in the urine as urea. The physiological fuel values were calculated as follows:

1.0 gram of carbohydrates = 17.46 × 0.98 = 16.27 MJ

1 gram of fat = 39.33 × 0.95 = 37.36 MJ

1 gram of protein = 23.64 – 5.25 × 0.92 = 16.00 MJ

The factor 5.22 MJ is too low to estimate the urine loss in case of herbivore because of excretion of large amount of hippuric acid instead of urea. Physiological fuel values are not applicable in case of ruminants because the digestibility of nutrient is low in ruminant than non-ruminants. Physiological fuel values are similar to metabolizable energy.

Q.1. Fill in the blanks.

1. The percent TDN = – – – – – – – – + – – – – – – + – – – – – + – – – – – – -

2. Only the losses in – – – is accounted in TDN system.

3. The percent ether extract content is multiplied by a factor – – – – in TDN system.

4. The term starch equivalent is given by – – – – – – – – .

5. In starch equivalent system – – – – – is taken as the net energy unit.

6. One Kg of digestible protein produces – – – – – g of fat.

7. One Kg of digestible starch produces – – – – – – g of fat when fed above the maintenance requirement.

8. The starch equivalent for one part digestible protein is – – – – – – – .

9. The starch equivalent for one part digestible fat is – – – – – – – – – .

10. The percentage of crude fibre to multiplied by the factor – – – – – to calculate corrected SE for dry roughages.

11. One Joule is equal to – – – – – – – calorie.

12. The joule is defined as – – – – – – – – – – – – – – .

13. Digestible energy is that portion of the gross energy of a feed which does not appear in the – – – – – – – – – .

14. Digestible energy includes — — — — — — — — and — — —
    — — — — — — —.

15. In Scandinavian Feed unit — — — — is taken as standard.

16. — — — — — — — — — built an apparatus for energy metabo-
    lism studies for farm animals.

17. The respiratory quotient (RQ) is the ratio — — — — — — —
    — — — — — — — — — —.

18. When carbohydrates are being oxidized in the body for
    energy purposes the RQ value is — — — — — —, whereas
    for fat and protein it is — — — — — — — and — — — — — —,
    respectively.

19. Physiological fuel value is a product of calorific value to
    its — — — — —.

20. Digestible nutrient namely — — — — — — is not added to
    calculate the TDN value.

21. — — — — — — — is used by animal to meet its maintenance
    requirement and to form new body tissues or products.

22. For an animal species, losses of energy in urine and meth-
    ane are relatively constant and are about — — — — — per-
    cent of D.E.

23. Gross energy (MJ /Kg DM) of carbohydrate, protein, fat
    and average foods are ...., — — — — — — — , — —
    — — — — — and — — — — — — respectively.

24. The original source of energy is ....

25. In brouwer equation, H.P.= — — — — — — — — — — — — — —
    — — — — — — — — — — — — —.

26. Direct calorimetry involves the feature of both — — — —
    — — — — and — — — — — — — —.

27. Indirect calorimetry needed only — — — — — because only
    — — — — — — — is recorded.

28. Portion of ME used for work, growth and milk produc-
    tion is called — — — — — — —.

29. ME is measured easily than DE in poultry because — — —
    — — — — — — and — — — — — — — are voided together.

Q.2. Explain the following.

1. How will you calculate TDN value and SE value of a feed?
2. Define the term energy, calorie and joule.
3. Explain the partitioning of food energy into its components.
4. Explain the direct calorimetery.
5. Explain the carbon- nitrogen balance method and Respiratory Quotient method for energy production.
6. Explain the gross energy, digestible energy, metabolizable energy, not energy, heat of increment and physiological fuel value.
7. Why digestible protein is also added to calculate TDN value inspite the protein is not a source of energy in normal condition?
8. Explain the factors affecting the TDN value and metabolisable energy value of a feed.
9. Explain associative effect of feed.

Evaluation of Protein Value of Feed in Animal Nutrition

It has long been known that all animals must receive in their food at least a certain minimum amount of protein. For simple stomach animals, the quality or kind of protein is fully as important as the amount. Fortunately, ruminant has much more simple requirement for protein than non-ruminants. This is because the rumen micro-organisms are able to use very simple nitrogen compounds as a protein source. This microbial protein is used by the ruminants. Different approaches to the evaluation of protein sources are therefore necessary for ruminant and non-ruminant animals.

Crude Protein (CP): Crude protein in the feed stuffs is estimated by determining the nitrogen content of feed and multiplying it by a factor 6.25. Two assumptions are made in calculating the protein content from the nitrogen: firstly, that all the nitrogen of the food is present as protein and secondly that all food protein contains 16g N/100g. The nitrogen content of the food is then expressed in term of crude protein (CP) calculated as follows.

CP (g/100g) = g nitrogen /100g × 100/16   Or more commonly

CP (g/100g) = g nitrogen /100g × 6.25

Both above assumptions are unsound. Different food proteins have different nitrogen contents, and therefore different factors should be used in the conversion of nitrogen for individual food. The nitrogen content of a number of common proteins together with appropriate nitrogen conversion factor is shown as:

Food protein	Nitrogen (g/100g)	Conversion factor
Cotton seed	18.87	5.30
Soyabean	17.51	5.71
Barely	17.15	5.83
Oat	17.15	5.83
Wheat	17.15	5.83
Maize	16.00	6.25
Egg	16.00	6.25
Meat	16.00	6.25
Milk	15.68	6.38

True Protein (TP): The term true protein is used to denote the protein only. It can be separated from non-protein nitrogen by precipitation with cupric hydroxide or by heat coagulation. The protein is then filtered and residue subjected to nitrogen estimation by Kjeldahl method. The protein is determined by multiplied the factor 6.25.

Digestible Crude Protein (DCP): When the crude protein content of the feed stuffs is multiplied by its digestibility coefficient, it gives the digestible crude protein. It is the most common way of expressing the protein values and requirement of the ruminants on most of the countries. In India, DCP is taken as the measure for expressing the protein values of feeds for ruminants. Digestible crude protein figures are not entirely satisfactory assessments of protein, because the efficiency with which the absorbed protein is used differs considerably from one source to another.

Protein Equivalent (PE): In some of the European countries protein equivalent is used instead of DCP. In protein equivalent non-protein nitrogen fraction is given half the nutritive of the true protein and is calculated as follows:

$$PE = \frac{\%DCP + \% DTP}{2}$$

So PE is the arithmetic mean of the percentage of DCP and DTP.

Protein Quality (PQ): In ruminants protein quality is not given much of the importance since all the essential amino acids are synthesized in the rumen by the synthesis of microbial proteins. However, digestible crude protein value for non-ruminant animal is not adequate to express the protein value. It is important to know how much of the absorbed protein is used by the animal body. This utilization will be different with the various protein sources as it is dependent upon the amino acid composition of the protein.

Evaluation of protein value of feed in non-ruminants:

Protein Efficiency Ratio (PER): The protein efficiency ratio normally uses growth of the rat as a measure of the nutritive value of dietary protein. It is defined as the weight gain per unit weight of protein eaten, and may be calculated by the following formula.

$$\text{Protein efficiency ratio} = \frac{\text{Gain in body weight (g)}}{\text{Protein consumed (g)}}$$

The PER values will vary with different protein sources as the composition of protein varies with regard to essential amino acids. For the optimum rate of growth, various level of protein would be required depending upon the quality. On this basis comparison between different sources of protein can be made. It is simplest method for evaluating protein quality.

Net Protein Retention (NPR) : A modification of PER method, where the weight gain of the experimental group is compared with a group on a protein free diet, give the net protein retention which is calculated as follows:

$$\text{NPR} = \frac{\text{Weight gain of test protein group fed - Weight loss of non-protein group fed}}{\text{Weight of protein consumed}}$$

The NPR method is claim to give more accurate results than the PER method.

Gross Protein Value (GPV): The body weight gain of chicks receiving a basal diet containing 8.0 g CP/100g are compared with those of chicks receiving the basal diet plus 3g/100 g of test protein, and of others receiving the basal diet plus 3 g /100 g of casein. The extra live weight gain per unit of supplementary test protein, stated as a proportion of the extra live weight gain per unit of supplementary casein, is the gross protein value of the test protein.

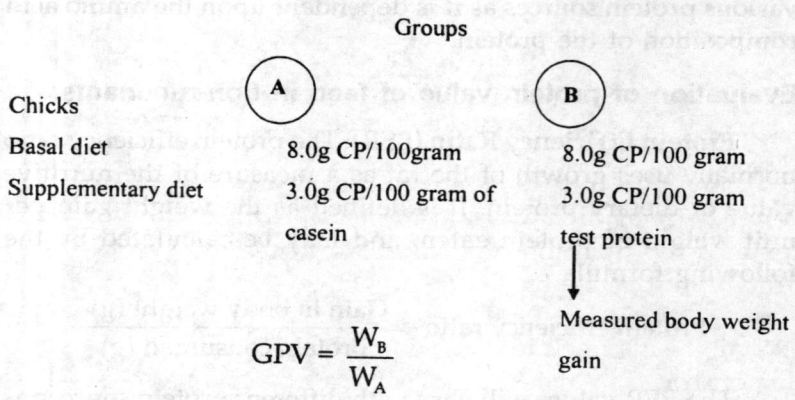

Groups

Chicks	A	B
Basal diet	8.0g CP/100gram	8.0g CP/100 gram
Supplementary diet	3.0g CP/100 gram of casein	3.0g CP/100 gram test protein

$$GPV = \frac{W_B}{W_A}$$

Measured body weight gain

where W_B is gram increased weight gain/gram of test protein and W_A is gram increase weight gain/g casein.

Protein Replacement Value (PRV): It is based on the nitrogen balance. This value measures the level at which the protein under test gives the same balance as an equal amount of standard protein. To evaluate the protein replacement value, two nitrogen balance studies are conducted; one for the standard protein likes egg or milk and another for the protein under test. The following equation is used for calculation of PRV.

$$PRV = \frac{A-B}{N \text{ intake}}$$

Where A = Nitrogen balance for standard protein in mg per basal K cal,

B = N balance for protein under test in mg per basal K cal.

The PRV measures the efficiency of utilization of the protein given to the animal. Other methods measure the utilization of digested and absorbed protein.

Biological Value (BV) of Proteins: It is defined as the proportion of nitrogen absorbed which is retained by the animals for maintenance and/or growth or proportion of digested protein that is not excreted in urine. A balance trial is conducted in which nitrogen intake and urinary and faecal excretions of nitrogen are measured, and the results are used to calculate the biological value as follows.

$$BV = \frac{N\ intake - (Faecal\ N + Urinary\ N)}{N\ intake - faecal\ N} \times 100$$

Part of the nitrogen in faeces, the metabolic faecal nitrogen, is not derived directly from the feed. Urinary nitrogen also contains a proportion of nitrogen, known as the endogenous urinary nitrogen, which is not directly derived from feed. The existence of nitrogen fractions in both faeces and urine whose excretion is independent of feed nitrogen is most conveniently demonstrated by the fact that some nitrogen is excreted when the animal is given a nitrogen free diet. It is obvious that their exclusion from the faecal and urinary fractions in the formula given above will give more precise estimate of biological value by Thomas- Mitchell formula.

$$BV = \frac{N\ intake - (Faecal\ N - MFN) - (urinary\ N - EUN)}{N\ intake - (Faecal\ N - MFN)}$$

where, MFN = Metabolic faecal nitrogen

EUN = endogenous urinary nitrogen.

The biological values of some of the proteins source have been given below:

Food	BV
Milk	95
Whole egg	94
Fish meal	74-89
Wheat	67
Maize	49-61
Soyabean meal	63-76
Cotton seed meal	63
Linseed meal	61
Barley	57-71
Peas	62-65

The biological values are dependent on the amino acid composition. If all the essential amino acid present in right amount and proportion than BV will be higher since the protein will be utilized for body tissues rather than being diverted for energy supply. In the latter case the amino acid will be deaminated and there will be more excretion of urea. Animal proteins have higher BV since the essential amino acids present in them are very near to the proportion in which they are needed by the body. Deficiency or excess of any one of the amino acids lowers the biological value.

Biological value of individual protein has a limited scope in practical feeding since no single protein is fed. Mixture of protein will have different biological value as it would not be a simple mean because one protein deficient in one amino acid may be supplemented by the addition of other. The biological values are also dependent on the level at which protein is being fed. It is maximum at maintenance level. For determining the B.V. the protein under test must be fed adequately as per requirement. Excess protein will reduce the BV. Adequate amount of energy must also be present in the diet otherwise protein would be used for energy purpose which would reduce the biological value of test protein.

Nitrogen balance: It evaluate protein quality in ruminants and non ruminants.

Nitrogen balance index: It is same as biological value.

$$NBI = \frac{\text{Nitrogen balance (B) - Nitrogen balance when N-intake is zero } (B_0)}{\text{Nitrogen absorbed}}$$

Net Protein Utilization (NPU): The usefulness of a protein to an animal will depend upon its digestibility as well as its biological value. The product of these two values is the proportion of the nitrogen intake which is retained, and is termed as the net protein utilization. It is based on comparison of body nitrogen content resulting from a test protein with that resulting over the same period on a nitrogen free diet.

$$NPU = \frac{\text{Body N. Content with test protein - Body N content with N free diet}}{\text{N intake}}$$

Or

$$NPU = \frac{\text{Retained Nitrogen}}{\text{Nitrogen intake}} \times 100$$

Net Protein Values (NPV): The product of the NPU and the percent crude protein is the net protein value (NPV) f the food, and is a measure of the protein actually available for metabolism by the animals.

Chemical score: Chemical score was given by Block & Mitchell (1946). There are methods in which protein quality is estimated without conducting the animal experimentation. The protein quality is dependent upon the amount and proportion of essential amino acids present in the protein. The value would be lower if one or more essential amino acids are deficient. The biological value of egg protein is higher since essential amino acids are present in right amount and proportion. In the chemical score method the content of each essential amino acids of a protein is determined and expressed as the percentage of standard and the lowest percentage is taken as the score. For example, in wheat protein lysine is the first limiting amino acid. The content of it is 7.2 and 2.7 percent in egg and wheat protein, respectively.

Amino Acids	Egg (%)	Wheat Protein (%)
Lysine	7.2	2.7
Isoleucine	8.0	3.6
Methionine	4.1	2.5

The chemical score for wheat protein is

$$\frac{2.7}{7.2} \times 100 = 37.0$$

These values compare with the biological values for protein in rat, pig and human being but not in poultry. It is because there are other amino acids which are deficient in the protein and are taken into account.

The Essential Amino Acids Index (EAAI): It was given by B.L. Oser (1951). In this case all the ten essential amino acids are considered. It is defined as the geometric mean of the egg ratio's of these acids to the food amino acids and may be calculated as follows:

$$EAAI = \sqrt[n]{\frac{a}{a_e} \times \frac{b}{b_e} \times \frac{c}{c_e} \times \frac{d}{d_e} \times \frac{j}{J_e}}$$

Where a, b..... J = concentrations g/100 gram of the essential amino acids in the food protein.

a_e, b_e..., ..., J_e = concentration of same amino acid in egg protein,

and n= the number of amino acids.

It has the advantage that all the essential amino acids are considered but proteins having different amino acids composition may have the same index.

Both the chemical score and the essential amino acid index are based upon gross amino acid composition. A more logical approach would be to use figure for the amino acids available to the animal.

Measures of Protein Quality in Practical Feeding of Pig and Poultry: The difficulties in assessing the value of proteins in the diet will now be apparent from the variety of methods that have been proposed, all of which have considerable limitations. A crude protein figure is useful, because the degradability of the proteins in foods commonly given to pig and poultry is fairly constant. More recently DCP has been used.

In practice pigs and poultry diets are based largely on cereals and assessment of the protein value of foods for such animals is then a question of measuring their ability to supplement the amino acid deficiencies of the cereals. To gross protein value is probably the most commonly used biological method for evaluating proteins.

Protein Quality for Ruminants: The significance of protein quality in ruminants is very limited since all the essential amino acids are synthesized by the micro-organism. The poor quality protein are improved in BV whereas, high quality proteins are degraded. The BV of microbial protein is about 70 but the overall BV of the food protein is very much less because of the production of ammonia in the rumen. Therefore, BV in the ruminants has little application.

For higher production, protein quality in ruminant is also getting importance. It has now being established that the microbial protein synthesized in the rumen are deficient in sulphur containing amino acid for higher production and specially for wool production in sheep in which cystine is present to the extent of 11 percent in the protein. Good quality protein should be protected from rumen degradation so that better amino acid mixture is available in the blood pool of the animals. The protection of protein is being done by physical means (heat treatment) or by chemical means of treating the protein with formaldehyde and tannic acid. Several alternative systems for evaluating the protein values in ruminants have been proposed.

1. Metabolisable protein: Metabolisable protein is that part of the dietary protein which is absorbed by the host animal and is available for use at tissue level. It consists partly of dietary true protein which has escaped degradation in the rumen but has been broken down to amino acid which are subsequently absorbed from the small intestine. Microbial protein synthesized in the rumen, similarly contributes to metabolisable protein. This system is used in the United State of America. Calculation of metabolisable protein schematically is given as:

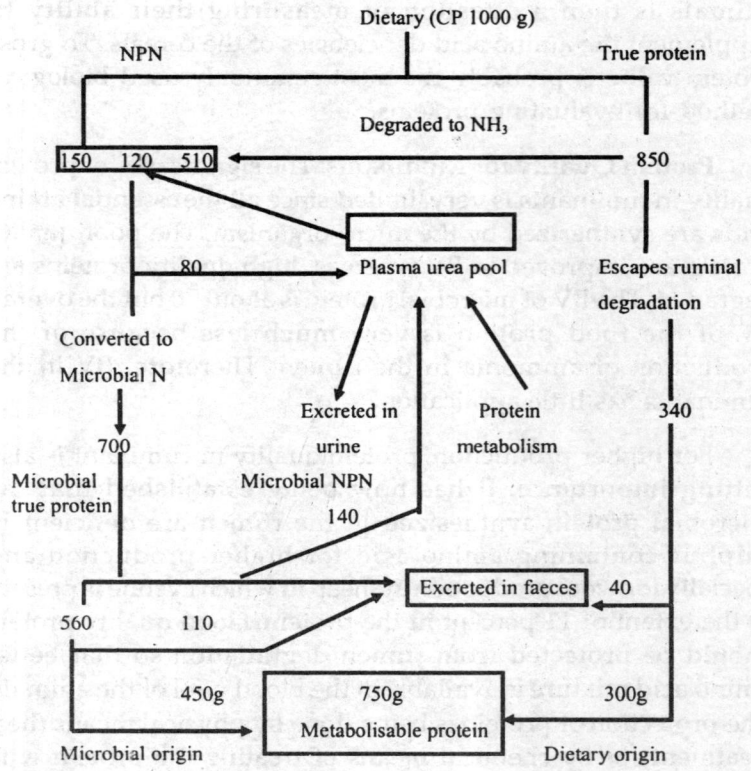

Calculation of metabolisable protein of diet.

2. Rumen degradable and undegradable protein: In this system of protein allowances, proposed by the Agricultural Research Council (ARC) for the United Kingdom and based on rumen degradable protein, i.e. that available to the microorganism, and undegradable protein which escapes degradation in the rumen but which undergoes digestion and absorption in the lower gut, and utilisation at tissue level.

The proportion of protein escaping breakdown in the rumen may be estimated in vivo by measuring dietary nitrogen intake, and non ammonia nitrogen and microbial nitrogen passing the duodenum. Degradability of nitrogen is then expressed as:

$$\text{Degradability} = 1 - \frac{\text{Non-ammonia duodenal N-Microbial N}}{\text{Dietary N intake}}$$

The duodenal nitrogen fraction contains microbial N and endogenous N. Microbial – N in duodenal –N is usually identified by means of marker substances such as diamino pimelic acid (DAPA), Amino ethyl phosphoric acid (AEPA), RNA, ^{35}S, ^{32}P and ^{15}N levelled amino acid.

The formula for calculating degradability given above ignores the fact that duodenal nitrogen contains a significant fraction which is of endogenous origin. It would be more accurate if degradability was calculated as follows.

$$\text{Degradability} = 1 - \frac{\text{Non-ammonia duodenal N-(Microbial N-Endogenous N)}}{\text{Dietary N intake}}$$

The endogenous N fractions constitute about 50 to 200 g/kg of duodenal nitrogen but are difficult to quantify.

A method of estimating protein degradation in the rumen by incubation of the food in synthetic fibre bag suspended in the rumen has been proposed. The degradability figure is calculated as the difference between the nitrogen initially present in the bag and that present after incubation, stated as a proportion of the initial nitrogen.

$$\text{Degradability} = \frac{\text{nitrogen - Nitrogen after incubation}}{\text{Initial nitrogen}}$$

The technique is subject to several source of error like sample size, bag size and porosity of the bag materials which must be controlled if reproducible results are to be obtained.

Q.1. Fill in the blanks:

1. The nitrogen content of a feed is multiplied by a factor – – – – – – – to calculate the protein content of that feed.

2. The conversion factor for milk nitrogen to convert it into protein content is – – – – – –.

3. Cotton seed protein contains – – – – – – percent nitrogen. So conversion factor for it – – – – – – –.

4. Protein equivalent is the — — — — — — — mean of the percentage of DCP and DTP.

5. Protein efficiency ratio is the weight gain per unit of — — — — — — — .

6. Net protein retention is a modification of — — — — — — — method.

7. Gross protein value calculation requires a basal diet containing — — — — — — — percent protein.

8. Biological value is the proportion of — — — — — — which is retained by the animals.

9. The biological value of milk protein is — — — — — — — — — .

10. The product of biological value of a protein to its digestibility Coefficient is called.

11. — — — — — — — and — — — — — — are the methods in which protein quality is estimated without conducting the animal experimentation.

12. In essential amino acid index method, — — — — — — — amino acids are considered.

13. The essential amino acid index is defined as the — — — — — — amino acids.

14. The proportion of dietary protein which escapes degradation in the rumen is called — — — — — — — — — .

15. Two assumptions for estimating protein content are, all nitrogen of food present in — — — — — — — and food protein contains — — — — — — — — — N/kg.

16. Animal protein has higher — — — value than plant protein.

17. Biological value is dependent primarily upon — — — — — .

18. Ideal protein is used for evaluating proteins for — — — — — — — .

19. For poultry, evaluation of protein source is based on — — — — — , — — — — and — — — amino acids.

20. — — — — — — — , — — — — — and — — — — — are used as growth response for protein in experimental animals especially monogastric animals.

21. $------$ and $-------$ are based on the proportion of main limiting amino acid of the protein.

22. The geometric mean of egg ratio's of these acids to the food amino acids is .called as $-------$.

23. Egg and wheat protein contains $--$ and $---$ percent lysine content,   respectively.

24. The product of NPU and percent CP is $--------$ $----$.

25. Gross protein value is defined as $------------$ $-----------------$.

26. The full form of DAPA and AEPA is $----------$ $----$and $------------$.

27. The duodenal nitrogen contains $----------$ and $--------------$.

28. Mixture of protein has $------------$ biological value.

Q.2. Explain the following.

Crude protein, True Protein, Non- Protein Nitrogen, Digestible crude protein, Protein equivalent, protein Efficiency ratio, Net protein retention, Gross protein value, Protein replacement value, Biological value, Net protein utilization, Net protein value, chemical score, Essential amino acid index, Metabolisable protein, Rumen degradable and undegradable protein.

Chapter 5

Processing Methods of Animal Feed Stuffs

Animal Feed technology: It deals with processing of feeds, fodders and preparation of formula feeds for which the knowledge of nutritional requirements of various livestock and poultry, quality control of feed ingredients, feed plant management and storage of feed ingredients and feeds are essential. It may also be defined as the application of physical, chemical, biochemical, biological, physiochemical and engineering methods to increase the nutrient utilization of feeds and fodders in animal system for the development of livestock and poultry and feed industry.

Objective of feed processing:

1. To make the feed more palatable.
2. To detoxify or remove undesirable ingredients
3. To make the storage easy and safe.
4. To increase nutrient content and nutrient availability.
5. To change the particle size or density of feed.
6. To make the animal production more economical.

Roughage processing methods: All these methods are broadly divided into two groups i.e. Dry processing method and wet processing method based on the addition or deduction of water content of roughages. These methods are further classified based on thermal treatment.

1. **Cold processing method:** It includes cracking/dry rolling, grinding, crimping, crumbling, extrusion, water soaking, reconstitution and decortication.

2. **Hot processing method:** It includes steam rolling, steam flaking, pressure cooking, exploding, gelatinization, popping, pelleting, roasting and micronizing.

    A.   **Dry processing methods:** In these methods water content is reduced to a desired level. It includes baling, field chopped, grinding, pelleting, cubing and dehydration.

1. **Baling:** The forage is cut and dried in the field condition. Dried forage is then baled or bundled. By this method we make storage and handling of forage easy and convenient.

2. **Chopping:** It is also known as chaffing. The forages are chopped into small pieces as fine or coarse particles. Chopping avoids the selective feeding thus wastage of plant material is reduced. The machine used for the intended purpose is called chaff cutter. Chopping facilitates easy handling due to increased bulk density and also improves digestion due to exposure of relatively large surface area of roughages for microbial digestion.

3. **Grinding:** It is a process of particle size reduction. Grinding of roughages improves the feed consumption and growth rate but reduces the digestibility of crude fibre due to faster rate of feed particles in gastro intestinal tract due to smaller particle size. But due to large cost, grinding of roughages is not economical.

4. **Pelleting:** The ground roughages are pelleted and fed to animals. It improves the consumption of poor quality roughages. A complete feed is made by pelleting poor quality roughage with 30 per cent concentrates. The size of pellets is 12 / 64" to 48/64" and has a density of 40 lb/cft whereas long hay roughages have density equal to 5 lb/cft.

5. **Dehydration:** It is a process of reduction of moisture content in a dehydrator using a temp. 600-1500°F for a short time period of 3-5 minutes. The dehydrated forage retains a lot of dry matter and protein and there is no loss of leaves, but carotene content is reduced due to dehydration.

6. **Cubbing:** It is a process of cub making. It increases the density of roughages upto 30 lb/cft. The good quality hay is sprayed with water to increase the moisture content upto 14 per cent and broken down rather than to ground the roughage so that there is minimum of fine particles in the cube.

B. **Wet processing method:** It includes soaking and green chopping. Soaking is a process of mixing or spraying water on roughages so that stems become soft and mixing of concentrates with roughage is uniform which improves the feed intake and digestibility of roughages. When green roughages are chaffed, there is no need of soaking and fed as such or mixed with dry roughage or concentrate mixture.

Processing of grains: Processing methods for grain are broadly divided into two groups as:

A. **Wet processing methods.** It includes soaking, steam rolling, flaking, pressure cooking, exploding, pelleting and reconstitution, extrusion, gelatinization.

B. **Dry processing methods:** It includes grinding, dry rolling, popping, micronizing, extruding and roasting, decorticating / dehulling, crimping and crumbling.

1. **Soaking:** Grains are soaked in water for 6 to 24 hours. The soaking softens the grains, which swells during the process and thus a palatable product is made. Soaked grains are easily mixed with roughages and wastage is reduced. Some time when soaked cakes of mustard and neem seed are filtered, help to remove the toxic factors present in cakes.

2. **Reconstitution:** It is similar to soaking water is added to mature dry grain to raise the moisture content to 25 to 30 percent and stored the wet grain in an oxygen limiting silo for 14 to 21 days prior to feeding. It also increases the solubility of the grain protein.

3. **Steam rolling:** The grain is subjected to live steam for different periods of time depending upon the pressure used

prior to rolling. At atmospheric pressure, 100°C temperature and 16-20 per cent moisture containing grain is steamed for 8 to 20 minutes whereas at a pressure of 20 to 60 psi preconditioning, grain having a temperature of 121 to 150°C and 18-25 percent moisture is steamed for a period of 1 to 2 minutes only. This only softens the grains without any significant change in starch granules. The only advantage of steam rolling over dry rolling is the production of large particles with little fines.

4. **Steam flaking:** Steam treatment is given for 15 to 30 min. due to which moisture content in the grains rises to 18-20 per cent. After rolling of such grains, flakes are produced. This process ruptures the starch granules and improves physical texture, nutrient utilization and performance of the animals in most of the cases.

5. **Pressure cooking and flaking:** In this process the grains are first cooked under steam pressure, cooled to room temperature and then rolled. The product is more or less similar to steam flaked grains but the processing is much expensive. Grains are cooked with live steam at 50 psi for 1.5 min in air tight pressure chambers, which achieved a temperature of 300°F. When flakes are made, this temperature is reduced to 200°F and moisture content up to 20 percent by passing them through cooling and drying tower.

6. **Extrusion:** A process of cooking in which feeds are also expanded by the application of adequate pressure is known as extrusion. The main purpose of extrusion is the gelatinization of starch in grains or complete feeds. It is also used for the incorporation of urea in starchy feeds and for the control of pathogenic microorganisms in the feeds of animal source.

7. **Exploding:** The process of swelling of steam treated grains under high pressure and sudden expose to atmospheric pressure or the grains are treated with high pressure steam (250 psi) for 20 seconds followed by sudden decrease to atmospheric pressure is known as exploding. It is done in steel vessel fitted with valve for injecting steam to raise

pressure inside the grain containing vessel to 250 psi for about 20 sec. After that outlet is opened through which treated grains escape in the shape of expanded grains with the husk removed. This happens due to entry of large amount of moisture in the kernels due to high pressure.

8. **Pelleting:** The process of densification of a ground grain or composite feed with or without the application of steam or moisture is known as pelleting. The ground feed material is forced to pass through the holes of specific size by a mechanical process. The machine used for the purpose is called pelleting machine. The purpose of pelleting is to change dusty and unpalatable feed material into more palatable, easy to handle large particles by application of optimum amount of heat, moisture and pressure. The normal size of pellets is 3.9 mm to 19 mm with cylindrical shape.

9. **Gelatinization:** The complete disintegration of starch granules of a grain brought about by the combined application of moisture, heat and pressure is known as gelatinization. It improves the digestion of feed by increasing water absorption ability and rate of action of amylase on soluble carbohydrates (starches).

Dry processing methods:

1. **Cracking or dry rolling:** It is the disintegration of kernels into particles with the application of pressure by moving rollers. It is done by a combination of breaking and crushing of the grains. The physical properties of dry rolled or cracked grain would be very similar to that of grains coarsely ground in a hammer mill.

2. **Crimping:** The process of rolling of feed ingredients with the use of corrugated rollers is called crimping. The process may include conditioning and cooling of the processed feed.

3. **Crumbles:** The feed of granular particle size produced from the grinding of pelleted feeds is called crumbles.

4. **Popping/puffing:** It is produced by the action of dry heat (370-425°C) for 15-30 seconds causing a sudden expansion

of the grain which rupture the endosperm and this results in rupture of starch granules and makes the starch more available to the animals. About 3 percent moisture of grain is lost during heat treatment. Popping reduces the density of grains and increases palatability and digestibility of starch. Popped grains are also a good carrier for molasses.

5. **Micronizing:** The popping of grains with the application of infra red heat energy having wavelength of 3×10^8 to 3×10^{11} cycles/second is called micronizing.

6. **Roasting:** The treatment of grains with direct flame is called roasting. It causes expansion in volume due to heating and generally increases digestibility. Roasting of whole soyabeans inactivates enzymes or inhibitory factors which improves the nutritive value for poultry.

7. **Grinding:** The process of reduction of feeds into particles with the application of pressure and shearing. It is a prerequisite for mixing, pelleting or extrusion. It is simplest and least expensive method which is accomplished with the help of hand stone mill, hammer mill and roller mills. The size distribution of grains depends on the shape, size and hardness of the kernel.

Advantages of grinding:

1. It is prerequisite for mixing, pelleting or extrusion.

2. It increases the surface area of grains which is reflected as improve feed utilization, digestibility and performance of animals.

3. It avoids selective feeding of grains and reduces the scope of shorting out less palatable feeds by the animals from the compounded mash.

4. Grinding increases compactness and reduces space requirement for storage.

Q.1. Fill in the blanks.

1. Chopping is also known as — — — — — — —.

2. In grinding the particle size of grain is — — — — — — — —.

3.   The density in pelleted feed is — — — — — — — — — —.
4.   Dehydration is a process of reduction of moisture content in a dehydrator using a temp. — — — — — — — for — — — — — — — minutes.
5.   Cubbing increases the density of roughages upto — — — — — — —.
6.   In soaking grain are soaked in water for — — — — — — — — hours.
7.   In reconstitution the moisture content of grain is raised upto — — — — — — —.
8.   The wet grains are stored in an oxygen limiting silo for 14 to 21 days prior to animal feeding in a process called — — — — — — — — — —.
9.   In steam flaking steam treatment is given for — — — — — — — minutes due to which moisture content in the grains rises upto — — — — — — percent.
10.   A process of cooking in which feeds are also expanded by the application of adequate pressure is known as — — — — — — — — — — —.
11.   The process of swelling of steam treated grains under pressure caused by the release to atmosphere is known as — — — — — — — — — —.
12.   The normal size of pellets is — — — — — — — — —.
13.   The complete disintegration of starch granules of a grain brought about by the combined application of moisture, heat and pressure is known as — — —.
14.   The process of rolling of feed ingredients with the use of corrugated rollers is called — — — — — — — — —.
15.   The feed of granular particle size produced from the grinding of pelleted feeds is called — — — — — — — — — —.
16.   The popping of grains with the application of infra red heat energy is called — — — — — — —.
17.   The treatment of grains with direct flame is called — — — — — — — —.

18. The process of reduction of feeds into particles with the application of pressure and shearing is called — — — — — — — — —.

19. Roasting of whole soybean inactivates enzymes which improves the nutritive value for — — — — — — — — — — — — — — — — —.

20. The size distribution of grains depends on — — — — — — — — — and — — — — — — — — —.

21. About — — — — — percent moisture of grains is lost during heat treatments.

22. The normal size of pellets is — — — — — to — — — — — with cylindrical shape.

23. Popping, micronizing and grinding are — — — — — — — — — — — — methods.

Q.2. Explain the following.

1. Dry processing methods for roughages.
2. Wet processing methods for roughages.
3. Wet processing methods for grains.
4. Dry processing methods for grains.
5. Objective of feed processing.
6. Define these terms: Baling, Chopping, Grinding, Pelleting, Dehydration, Cubbing, Soaking, Reconstitution, Steam rolling, Steam flaking, Pressure cooking, Extrusion, Exploding, Gelatinization, Cracking or dry rolling, Crimping, Crumbles, Popping, Micronizing, Roasting,
7. Advantage of grinding and pelleting.

Various Feed Processing Methods for Improving the Nutritive Value of Inferior Quality Roughages

Feed accounts for 60-70 percent of total cost of livestock production. Inferior quality roughages are dry fibrous crop residues available for the feeding of livestock like wheat straw, paddy straw, finger millet straw and barley straw and stover (kadbi) of sorghum, pearl millet and maize etc. These straw and stovers are now considered as conventional dry roughages for the feeding of farm animals in India. Several non-conventional dry roughages are also used for the feeding of animals, which are sugar cane trash, baggase and fallen tree leaves etc. But due to low voluntary intake, low digestibility, low crude protein, essential minerals and vitamins content and presence of certain antinutritional factors like lignin, silica, oxalates and tannins make their utilization inefficient even by the ruminant animals. The situations manifest itself as poor animal performance, low growth rate, reduced fertility, high mortality and incidence of disease and parasitism. So there is a need for quality improvement of dry fibrous crop residues and other similar roughages. Various methods for improving the nutritive value of poor quality roughages are classified as-

Physical Treatment: Soaking, chopping, Grinding Pelleting, Wafering, Steam treatment and Irradiation.

Chemical treatment: Alkali treatment, Ammonia treatment, Acid treatment etc.

Biological treatment: Enzyme, rot fungi, mushroom and yeasts.

A. Physical treatment:

1. Supplementation with deficient nutrients source: Various nutrients are added by their enriched source to compensate the deficiency of that particular nutrient in poor quality straw. Addition of urea, molasses, green fodder, legume straw, ensiling straw with top feeds minerals and vitamins supplements are helpful to improve the nutritive value of poor quality straw for animals.

Molasses: Molasses is the by product of sugar industry. It contains about 45-50 percent sugar. Molasses has been mainly used in animal feeding at 5-10 percent level. These levels were mostly used as-

1.   Carrier for urea impregnation of poor quality roughages.
2.   As binder for commercial pelleted feeds for the convenients and economic feeding of livestock eg. uromol.
3.   As sweetener for increasing voluntary intake of compounded feed.

Now present time urea molasses mineral blocks (UMMB) are also used as supplements in animal feeding. At Ludhiana, Uromol compound was prepared by heating urea and molasses in the ratio of 9:1 (w/w) at 110°C.

2. Irradiation – Improvement of digestibility of wheat straw by high voltage X-rays has been found to be due to the breaking of the cellulose and hemicellulose bonds, resulting in formation of oligosaccharides. This can be utilized by rumen organisms. Forage lignin resists the X-rays. Upon irradiation ergosterol, a plant sterol yields calciferol, commonly known as vit. D_3. This method involves high cost and technology.

B. Chemical treatments:

The aim of chemical treatment is to breakdown the lignocellulose complex and the swelling of cell walls facilitates the easy access of rumen microbial enzymes to the cellulose and hemicellulose fraction of the feeding material. Various chemical treatments are explained as:

Acid treatment: The acid treatment changes the chemical composition to a certain extent without any alteration in the nutrient utilization. Various organic and inorganic acids may be used. But it is cost effective process and have low practical utility.

Treatment with oxidizing agents: Various oxidising agents like alkaline hydrogen peroxide, ozone, sulphur oxide, sodium sulphite and bleaching powder are effectively used to nutritional improvement of poor quality roughages. But due to high cost of treatment and lack of suitable technology for large scale treatment are the main limiting factors for this treatment.

Alkali treatment: Various alkalies like sodium hydroxide, lime, caustic soda, sodium bicarbonate and ammonia are used to improve the nutritive value of poor quality roughages which are explained below.

I. Sodium hydroxide treatment:

Wet treatment: The roughages are chopped and treated with 1.5 percent (W/V) NaOH solution for at least 4 hours. The treated straw was drained and washed with a large quantity of water to remove all the NaOH solution.

Dry treatment: In this treatment chaffed dry fodder is first spread on clean hard floor or thick plastic sheet. Solution of NaOH (3-4%) is sprinkled and mixed with fodder. 4 to 6 kg of NaOH dissolved in 200 litres of water is adequate to wet 100 kg fodder. This makes the fodder moist and has pleasant odour and improved nutritive value. But care should be taken to protect the skin from NaOH which is corrosive in nature. But cost of NaOH solution increase the cost of treatment, which is not economical in general, conditions. During the First World War (1914-18) a product "fodder cellulose" was produced in Germany by treating straw with NaOH under high pressure and high temperature.

2. Treatment with lime: Since calcium oxide and calcium

hydroxide are weak alkali, higher amount is required for longer duration for straw treatment. It is safe, economical and easily available chemicals than sodium hydroxide.

3. Ammonia treatment: Ammonia is also used to improve the nutritive value of straw. It serves as an alkali to potential rate and extent of digestion of straw and as a source of nitrogen for rumen microbes. In this treatment stacks of straw were wrapped with polyethylene cover and injected with 3% ammonia. Aqueous ammonia (20-35%) is also used for straw treatment.

4. Urea ammoniation treatment: It is the most convenient method of chemical treatment to straw. Urea is easily available and well known to farmers. In this method weighted chaffed straw is spread on the polythene sheet in a layer of 45-50 cm 3 kg urea is dissolved in 40 litres of water for 100 kg straw. The urea solution is sprayed over the straw, mixed uniformly and then stacked air tight and left for 3 weeks. After that stack is opened and straw is ready for animal feeding after overnight aeration of straw.

In order to reduce the loss of nitrogen during treatment of roughages tier system method is applied in which alternate layers of 3 per cent followed by 2 per cent urea treated roughages are stacked. The excess ammonia in higher concentration layer diffuses to the lower concentration layer and results in considerable saving of urea and ammonia. Sometime a top layer of about 20-30 cm. thickness acidified with mild solution of commercial sulphuric acid may be used. This layer absorbs large proportion of unutilized ammonia.

Conditions for urea treatment: For the better results, some conditions are to be maintained so that urea hydrolysis should be complete which are as:

Moisture level: 35-40 litres of water for 100 kg roughages is sufficient for ureolysis.

Temperature: The optimum temperature for urease activity in soil is $30^{\circ}C$. Ammoniation is increased at higher temperature.

Level of urea: Optimum level of urea should be used for better utilization as well as to avoid toxicity of urea. 4-5 percent urea (V/V) solution may be used. Urease enzyme is a natural contaminant of straw. Urea was extensively hydrolysed by this enzyme. But addition of an urease source reduces the treatment time. Soyabean powder (8.5%) is an urease source.

5. Treatment with animal urine: Animal urine an unconventional NPN source abundantly available is also used to improve the nutritive value of poor quality roughages.

Precautions for chemical treatments:

(i)   Mixing of the chemicals should be thorough and uniform.

(ii) Chemicals should be handled carefully as these are corrosive in nature.

(iii) Ammonia is an explosive in nature so fire should not be ignited near the stock or during the injection of ammonia gas.

(iv) Ammoniated fodders should be properly aerated before feeding to the animals.

(v)   Animals should be adapted to chemical treated roughages by feeding low concentrated chemical treated roughages initially.

C. Biological treatment: Biological treatments involves the living organisms specially microbes (Fungi) to improve the nutritive value of poor quality roughages. In this treatment poor quality straws are treated with aerobic fungi namely white rot fungi such as *Sporotrichum* sp., *Lenzitis* sp., *Coprinus* sp. *Trichusus spiralis*, *Pacilomyces fusisporus* etc. Pure culture of fungus strain are raised on suitable medium and then incubated with straw at varying moisture level for different periods, which will improve the nutritive value of straw.

Most microorganisms have some effect on crop residues and other fibrous materials and metabolise lignin, cellulose and other fibrous components. They should have the ability to break down the ligno-cellulose complex and degradation of lignin and cellulose with their enzyme secretion. So that digestibility of these cell wall components may improve. The ideal microorganisms for biological treatment should have strong lignin metabolism with low or no affinity towards cellulose and hemicelluloses. The biological methods of straw treatment which involves the use of microorganisms capable of degrading lignin by producing extra cellular "*Phenol oxidase*" the enzyme which are probable involves in the process of lignin degradation and thus rendering cellulose and hemicellulose fraction free. A high activity cellulase is required for enzymatic hydrolysis of cellulose.

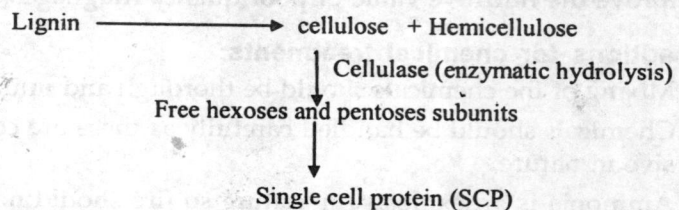

Free hexoses and pentoses subunits are used for single cell protein. Best results of Biological treatment are obtained when the roughage incubated with fungal spore for the period of at least 30 days. But care should be taken that these microbes should not produce toxins, easy to handle and cost effective. Thus, these methods have great appeal as an alternative to the use of expensive chemical and physical methods to produce economic ruminant feeds.

Q.1. Fill in the blanks.

1. Feed is the major input in livestock farming which accounts for ……….. percent of total cost of production.
2. Optimum level of molasses is ………… which is used in animal feeding.
3. Full form of UMMB……….. used in animal feeding.
4. In forage …………. resist the X-rays.
5. …………. and …………. are required for longer duration for straw treatment.
6. Animal urine is an unconventional …………. source.

7. The optimum level of urea ....% (v/v) solution is used for bette r utilization of poor quality roughages.

8. .... is an explosive in nature so fire should not be ignited near the stock.

9. Main fungi involved in biological treatment of roughages are ...., ... and ....

10. The fungi secrete an enzyme .... which degraded the lignin.

11. The phenol oxidase enzyme degrades the lignin into ...... fraction free.

12. Free hexoses and pentoses subunits are used in ....

13. Best result of biological treatment of roughages is obtained when it is incubated for a period of .... with fungal spore.

14. – – – – – – – enzyme is a natural contaminants of straw.

15. During First World War "fodder cellulose" was produced in Germany by treating – – – – – – – – with – – – – – under high pressure and temperature.

16. Molasses is used in commercial pelleted feed as – – – –.

17. Uromol is prepared by heating urea and molasses in the ratio of – – – – – – – (w/w) at 110^0 C.

18. Some common examples of poor quality roughages are – – – – – – – –, – – – – – – – – – – – –, – – – – – – – – – and – – – – – – – – –.

Q.2. Explain the following.

1. Various feed processing methods for improving the nutritive value of roughage.

2. Why lignin is degraded in roughages when it is treated with fungal spores.

3. Short notes on-

   a. Physical treatment of roughage.

   b. Chemical treatment of roughage.

   c. Biological treatment of roughage.

   d. Single cell protein

Chapter 7

Harmful Natural Constituents and Toxic Substances in Animal Feeds

A toxicant is a substance, which under practical circumstances can impair some aspect of animal metabolism and produce adverse biological or economical effects in animal production. This is a broad definition, but encompasses those aspects that are relevant in livestock production. Virtually everything is toxic, if given in large enough dose. Thus, the term "toxicant" refers only to those substances which might normally be encountered at toxic levels. Other terms used synonymously with toxicant are "poison" and "toxin".

Anti-nutritional factors may be defined as those substances in the diet which by themselves or their metabolic products arising in the system interfere with the feed utilization, reduced production or affects the health of the animals. Toxicants can be classified based on their chemical properties and their effect on utilization of nutrients.

1. According to their chemical properties:

1. Alkaloids - Pyrrolizidine and piperidine alkaloids.

2. Glycosides - Saponins, cyanogens, Glucosinolates.

3. Proteins - Protease inhibitors and Haemagglutinins.

4. Metal binding - Substance or inorganic toxicants.

5. Phenols - Gossypol and Tannins.

6. Mycotoxins

2. Effect on nutrient utilization

1. Substances affecting protein utilization are protease inhibitor, haemagglutinin, saponin and polyphenolic components.

2. Substances reducing solubility or interfering with the utilization of minerals are phytic acid, oxalic acid, gossypol and glucosinolates.

3. Substances affecting carbohydrates digestion are amylase inhibitors, phenolic compounds and flatulence factors.

4. Substances increasing the vitamins requirements.

1. Alkaloids: Alkaloids are basic substances that contain nitrogen in heterocyclic ring. They are widely distributed in the plants; it has been estimated that 15-20% of all vascular plants contain alkaloids. Most alkaloids are derived from amino acids in their synthesis by plants. Amino acids are decarboxylated to amines and the amines are converted to aldehydes by amine oxidase. Condensation of the aldehyde and amine groups then yields the heterocyclic ring. Various alkaloids with their sources are tabulated below

Alkaloids with their sources

Atropine	Deadly nightshade
Cocaine	Leaves of Coca plant
Coniine	Hemlock
Morphine	Dried latex of opium poppy
Nicotine	Tobacco
Quinine	Cinchona bark
Solanine	Unripe potatoes
Strychnine	Seeds of nux vomica

Pyrrolizidine alkaloids (PA) contain the pyrrolizidine nucleus. The structure of serecionine and heliotrine are representative of toxic principle in livestock nutrition. The PAs are biosynthesized from amino acids such as ornithine. Most of the PA containing plants used in livestock feeding are in the genera Senecio, Crotaliaria, Heliotropium and Echium. The principle pathology is irreversible liver cirrhosis with pronounced fibrosis and biliary hyperplacia. Mortality is related to impair liver function. The most important piperidine alkaloids in animal production are coniine and related alkaloids found in *Conium maculatum* (poison hemlock). These alkaloids affect the central nervous system and are also teratogens. An example of pyridine is nicotine in *Nicotiana* spp. (cultivation and wild tobacco).

Indoles are the derivatives of the amino acid tryptophane Examples are the ergot alkaloids such as perloline. The quinolizidine nucleus consists of two six-membered rings. Lupines contain these alkaloids which cause acute poisoning in sheep and teratogenic effect in calves (crooked calf disease). Tryptamine alkaloids are found in Phalaris tuberosa, a forage grass grown in Australia. Phalaris poisoning results in acute neurological sign and chronic muscular incordination. A tropine, found in Datura spp. (Jimson weed), is an example of a tropane alkaloid. It has pronounced effect on the central nervous system.

2. Glycosides: Glycosides are ethers containing a carbohydrate moiety and a non-carbohydrate moiety (aglycone) joined with an ether bond. They are usually bitter substances. Often the aglycone is released by enzymatic action when the plant tissue is damaged, as by wilting, freezing and mastication. They are classified on the basis of aglycone.

(a) Cyanogens: Cyanogens are glycosides of a sugar or sugars (usually glucose) and cyanide containing aglycone. They can be hydrolysed by enzymatic action with the release of hydrogen cyanide which is a potent toxin. The major cyanogens of importance in animal nutrition are the following.

(i)   Amygdalin (lactrile): This glycoside found in Rosaceae, such as chokecherries, wild cherries. Mountain mahogany and the kernels of almonds, apricots, peaches and apples. Prunasin is also found in these plants; it has the same structure as amgydalin except it has one glucose rather than two attached to the aglycone.

(ii) Dhurrin: This occurs in sorghum species such as grain sorghum, forage sorghum (sudan grass) and Johanson grass.

269

(iii) Linamarin: This compound is found in white-clover, flax (Lin seed), cassava and Lima beans.

Hydrogen cyanide is formed when the glucosides are hydrolyzed by plant enzymes (β-glucosidase and hydroxynitrilelyase).

Mode of action HCN: HCN is readily absorbed and enters in tissue cells. It affects the electron transport system at two sites by affecting the cytochrome oxidase.

(i) Cytochrome-b is reduced to lesser extent in the presence of cyanide.

(ii) The electron transfer from cytochrome-a to water is completely inhibited, ATP formation ceases and the tissues suffer energy deprivation and death follows rapidly.

In subacute conditions oxygen is not taken up by the tissue because blood does not transfer the oxygen. So that arterial blood remains like venous blood. In acute condition when the quantity eaten is more it paralyses the medula oblongata in brain where respiration receptors are located, therefore, respiration stops and leading to death.

Sign of HCN toxicity: Sign of cyanide poisoning are dyspnoea (difficult breathing), excitement, gasping, paralysis, staggering, convulsion, coma and death. Cyanide is readily detoxified. Liver, kidney and thyroid tissue contain an enzyme rhodanase which catalyzes conversion of cyanide to thiocyanate, which is excreted in the urine. Ammonia and nitrite inhalation is also useful during mild toxicity.

(b) Glucosinilates: Glucosinolates are glycosides of β-D-thioglucose with an aglycone that yields an isothiocyanate, nitrile or thiocyanate or similar structure upon hydrolysis. Most of the glucosinolate containing crucifers that are important in human or animal nutrition are in the genus Brassica includes cabbage, broccoli, rapeseed, mustard and turnips.

The glucosinolates are hydrolysed by an enzyme system (glucosinolase or thiglucosidase). The enzyme is found in plant and is released when the plant material is crushed. It is also produced by the rumen microorganisms. The major effect of the hydrolysis products of glucosinolates is inhibition of the function of thyroid gland and results in goitre. The thyroid produces hormone known as thyroxine that are important in regulating the rate of cellular metabolism.

Sign of glucosinolate toxicity: Goiter in humans has been observed. Poultry and swine fed raw rapeseed meal exhibited enlarge thyroid, growth depression, perosis, low egg production, off flavours in egg and liver damage.

Treatment:

1. Feeding of iodinized salt reduces the incidence in man and animals.

2. Heat treatment of rapeseed reduces the glucosinolate.

3. Thyroxine therapy may be useful for curing the disease.

(c) Coumarin: Sweet clover poisoning, sweet clover (*Melilotus albus* and *Melilotus officinalis*) contains a glycoside called melilotoside, an ether of glucose and coumarin. Coumarin is metabolised to produce dicoumarol. Dicoumarol is an inhibitor of vitamin K and induces a vitamin K deficiency which is characterized by susceptibility to haemorrhage.

Sweet clover poisoning occurs almost exclusively in cattle. The predominant sign is haermorrhage. Internal haermorrhage results in bovine subcutaneous swellings caused by pooling of blood. The mucous membranes are pale, and the animal becomes weaker and dies without struggle. Sweet clover poisoning can be treated with injections of vitamin K and whole blood transfusion.

(d) Saponins: Saponins are glycosides widely distributed among plants like chick-pea, soyabean, alfalfa and common beans. Saponins are characterized by a bitter taste and foaming properties and involved in bloat in ruminants. Saponins have industrial and commercial applications, including use in soft drinks, shampoo, soap and the synthesis of steriod hormones.

Pasture species that causes livestock problems because of their phytoestrogen content includes subclover, red clover and alfalfa. The estrogens in clovers are usually isoflavones, while alfalfa contains coumestans. Due to the action of micro-organism in rumen of sheep and cattle the isoflavones are converted into equol and phenolic acid.

Physioloigical effects of phytoestrogens: After sheep have grazed estrogenic for several years the fertility of the flock becomes depressed. The condition of permanent infertility is known as clover disease. The main cause of infertility is a failure of fertilization associated with poor sperm penetration to oviduct. The cervical mucous has an altered consistency which impairs sperm storage in the cervix. In ewes affected by clover disease, the cervix shows structural and functional changes. In sheep uterine prolaps, interference in sperm transportation in female, abnormal ova transport and uterine cyst have been noted.

Mechanism of action

1. Some results indicated that normal hormonal interrelationship is interefered resulting in failure of endogenous estrogens.

2. Pituitary seems to be achieving site because the pituitary basophils in ewes given coumestan diet is enlarged causing inhibition of gonadotropin releasing factor from the pituitary.

3. The depression in ovulation rate with coumestane diet also appears to be in some way related to FSH.

4. Folicular abnormalities in ovary have also been noticed in ewes given red clover.

3. Proteins and amino acids:

(i) **Trypsin (protease) inhibitors:** A wide variety of plants contain protein fraction which inhibit protein digestion in the digestive tract of animal. The trypsin inhibitors of soyabeans are the best known and most widely studied. Other plant containing trypsin inhibitors include most types of beans, potatoes, rye, triticale, barley and alfalfa. Protease inhibitior is probably a better term, since other enzymes such as chymotrypsin are also affected.

Nutritional significance of trypsin inhibitor: Soyabean is the major protein supplement used in swine and poultry diets. It must be heat treated to destory trypsin inhibitors. The mode of action of trypsin inhibitors is not entirely clear. In nonruminant includes poor growth, reduced feed intake, a reduction in protein digestibility, pancreatic hypertrophy and a deficiency if sulphur containing amino acids. Trypsin inhibitors are readily destroyed by treatment of plant material with heat. Over 95% of the activity is destroyed in 15 min. at 100°C.

(ii) Hemagglutinins (lectins): Hemagglutinins (*Phytohemagglutinins, lectins*) cause the clumping or agglutination of red blood cells in vitro. They were first isolated from castor beans, which contain a potent lectin called ricin. Lectins are proteins that have a high affinity for certain sugar molecules. Probably their biological effects are due to their affinity for sugars.

Lectins are found in soyabean and other field beans such as kidney, pinto and navy bean. Haemagglutinin causes various adverse effects, including reduced growth, diarrhoea, decreased nutrients absorption and increased incidence of bacterial infection. The major effects seem to be on the intestinal mucosa. In addition, there is evidence that lectins impair the immune system. Lectins are destroyed by moist heat. They are resistant to dry heat.

(iii) Bloat- producing proteins: Bloat is a distension of the rumen as a result of the inability of the animal to eructate gases produced in normal processes to rumen fermentation. The principle gases are carbondioxide and methane and these gases are trapped in the form of stable foam. The eructation mechanism is inhibited by the presence of foam at the base of the oesphagus; eructation of foam would result in it getting in to the lungs. Bloat producing plants, primarily legumes, contain substances which causes the production of a stable foam in the rumen. The most important bloating species in temperate regions are alfalfa (*Medicago sativa*), red clover (*Trifolium pratense*) and white clover (*T. repens*). Tropical legumes are not bloat producers. In addition, animal factors as well as rumen microbes are also involved in bloat condition. The use of antifoaming agents such as poloxalene (Bloat Guard) and vegetable oil in legume pastures has vastly reduced the bloat problems.

(iv) Mimosine: Subabul (*Leucaena leucocephala*), commonly referred to as leucaena, is a tropical legume with great potential as a protein source for livestock. It is vigorous, rapidly growing, drought tolerant, palatable, high yielding crop and its leaves contain 25-30% crude protein. These potential attributes are presently limited by the occurrence of the toxic amino acid mimosine in leucaena. Mimosine is structurally very similar to tyrosine and in rumen it is metabolized to 3,4 dihydroxypyridine (DHP). DHP is a goitrogen, impairing the incorporation of iodine in to iodinated compounds in the thyroid gland.

In non- ruminant mimosine causes poor growth, alopecia and eye cataracts. Ruminant animals may show various symptoms such as poor growth, loss of hair, swollen and rough coronets above the hooves, lameness, mouth and oesophageal lesions, depressed serum thyroxine level and goiter developed.

(v) Lathyrogens: Lathyrism is a crimpling disease in humans caused by the consumption of seeds of *Lathyrus* spp., principally *L. sativus (chick pea)*. Lathyrism is of two types: neurolathyrism and osteolathyrism.

Osteolathyrism: This is the principal form of lathyrism that affects livestock. Consumption of seeds of *L. odoratus, L. silvestris and L. hiscsutus*. The lathyrogen in *lathyrus odoratus* and related species is β- amino propionitrile (BAPN), an amino acid derivative. BAPN causes skeletal deformity and rupture due to defective synthesis of cartilage and connective tissue. Malformations of long bones are caused by irregular hyperplastic cartilage formed in the epiphysis. Arotic rupture due to the formation of arotic aneurysm, is due to defective collagen and elastin synthesis.

Neurolathyrism: Neurolathyrism is a paralysis of legs due to nerve damage in the spinal cord caused by neurotoxins in *L. sativus, L. latifolius* and *L. cevcera*. The principal neurolathyrogen is β-N- oxalye- L-α-β- diamino propionic acid (ODAPP).

4. Metal-binding substances and inorganic toxicants:

A. Oxalates: Oxalates of certain foods precipipate calcium in the gastrointestinal tract as insoluble calcium oxalate. Paddy straw and Pusa gaint Napier grass and some other green fodder and tree leaves are rich in oxalate. Oxalate containing feed causing a calcium deficiency in cattle resulting poor milk production and growth. Poultry are also affected. Animal response to oxalate poisoning varies with species of animals and plants.

B. Phytic acid: It is an ester formed by combination of the six alcoholic groups of inositol of with six molecules of hexaphosphoric acid. Seeds of cereals, dried legumes, oil seeds and nuts are rich in phytic acid. It depresses the utilization of several mineral elements such as phosphorus, calcium, magnesium, Iron and zinc etc. by forming the insoluble compounds, which are excreted in the faeces. Supplementation of enzyme phytase in poultry makes the phosphorus available for birds.

C. Minerals as toxicants: Though minerals are very essential for maintenance and growth for all animal species but their excess amount in diet may produce harmful effects. The selenium, molybdenum, fluorine, sulphur are few minerals which have significant toxic effect in animal production and health. Common salt, phosphorus and some other trace minerals have also adverse effect if consumed in excess amount.

5. Phenols:

(i) **Gossypol:** It is found in cotton seed. It is available in free form as a well bound form as gossypol-protein complex. Whole cotton seed contains 1.09-1.53 percent of gossypol. Heat treatment of Cotton seed meal decreases the gossypol content. The physiological effects of free gossypol are reduced appetite, loss of body wt., reduced heamoglobin content, cardiac irregularities, accumulation of fluid in body cavities and depress liver function. It is more toxic to non-ruminants than ruminants because in rumen gossypol combines with soluble protein. This complex is resistant to enzymatic break down. Gossypol also combines with Iron and lysine. So ferrous sulphate supplementation reduces the toxic effect of gossypol.

(ii) **Tannin:** It is a high molecular wt. polyphenolic substance widely distributed in nature. It is of two types i.e. hydrolysable tannins which can be readily hydrolysed by water, acids, bases or enzymes and yield gallotannins and ellagitannins. Condensed tannins are flavonoids- polymers of flavonol. Sorghum, salseed meal, mustard oil cake and lucerne meal contain sufficient amount of tannin.

Tannins are astringent in nature. They bind with protein and reduces its availability to animals. They depress cellulase activity and thus digestion of crude fibre reduces. Most of the tannins are present in seed coat. So decortication of seeds will decrease the tannin content. Other physical methods like soaking and cooking reduce the tannin content. Addition of tannin complexing agents like polyethylene glycol (PEG) and polyvinyl proldone (PVP) prevent formation of protein-tannin complex as well as break the already formed complex thus liberating protein.

6. **Mycotoxins:** Aflatoxins are a group of closely related toxic substances produced by the fungi, *Aspergillus flavus* and *Aspergillus parasiticus*, mostly in improperly stored feedstuffs such as cereal grains and oil meals. Although other fungi such as *Penicillium* spp, *Rhizopus* spp, *Muco* spp. and *Streptomyces* spp. are capable of producing aflatoxins, but their toxicity to livestock production has not been established. The name "aflatoxin" derives from- *Aspergillus* (a-), flavus (-fla-) and toxin. *A. flavus* and *A. parasiticus* produce four major toxins: B_1, B_2, G_1 and G_2. These were named according to their fluorescence properties under shortwave ultraviolet light on thin-layer chromatography. B_1 and B_2 fluoresce blue, whereas G_1 and G_2 fluoresce green. Fourteen other aflatoxins are known but most of these are

metabolites, formed endogenously in animals administered one or more of the four major aflatoxins. Metabolites of toxicological significance includes, aflatoxin B_1-2,3 oxide (AFB$_1$-2,2 oxide), aflatoxin M_1 (AFM$_1$); aflatoxicol and aflatoxin B_2 (ABF$_{2a}$).

Aflatoxins were first discovered as toxic factors when heavy mortality occurrred amongst turkeys, ducklings and patridges in early 1960 in England. The cause was known to be mycotoxins in mouldy groundnut meal that was imported from Brazil to England for the use as protein supplement in animal diets.

Aflatoxin-producing strains of *Aspergillus* are the constituents of microflora of air and the soil throughout the world. When environmental conditions are favourable, then colonization and mould growth can easily be occur on the substrate (feed or seed). Strain variations, nature of substrate and environmental conditions (temperature, moisture, aeration) influence the aflatoxin production with respect to their type and their individual concentrations. The relative humidity surrounding the substrate was the most improtant factor for the growth of *Aspergillus flavus*. Optimum temperature for alfatoxin production by *A. flavus* has been shown to be 25⁰C for aflatoxin B_1 and 30⁰C for G_1. *A. flavus* is primarily a seed-colonizing mould and is usually referred to as a storage mould. Three major feedstuffs with high potential for invasion by Aspergillus spp. during growth, harvest, transportation or storage are corn, cotton seed and groundnut (Peanut).

Effects of aflatoxin on productivity of animals:

Acute intoxication: Acute intoxication poisoning of farm animal is less likely to occur than chronic aflatoxicosis. The principle target organ in all species is the liver. Numerous liver functions are affected and the cumulative impact can be fatal to animals. Hepatocytes undergo progressive changes such as infilteration with lipids eventually ending in necrosis. These toxic effects are believed to be result of widespread and non-specific in interactions between AFB$_1$ or its metabolites and various cell proteins. Interaction with key enzymes can disrupt basic metabolic processes in the cell such as carbohydrates or lipid metabolism, and protein synthesis. Modification of permeability characteristics of hepatocytes or subcellular organelles, primarily the mitochondria, contributes to the necrosis. As the liver losses its functionality, other effects appear such as derangement of blood clotting mechanism (coagulopathy), icterus (jaundice), and reduction of essential serum proteins, which are synthesized in the liver.

In young swine, which are highly susceptible to acute poisoning, early hepatocytic changes occur within 6 hr. after exposure. Haemorrhages and cell necrosis occur by 9-12 hours, elevated serum glutamicoxalo-acetate transaminase (SGOT) at 12-14 hr, and death followed within 24-34 hr. In general, these same biological changes occur in all acutely intoxicated species. However, the susceptibility among different species is highly variable. Rabbits and ducks are highly sensitive to aflatoxins, whereas, sheep and rat are less sensitive.

Chronic intoxication: Chronic poisoning or aflatoxicosis can result when low levels of toxin are ingested over a prolonged period. In general, affected livestock exhibit decreased growth rate, lowered productivity (meat and eggs) and immuno suppression. Carcinogenicity has also been observed and studies in several species. Liver damage is also prevalent in chronic aflatoxicosis in all species. At necropsy, the liver is usually pale to yellow, and the gall bladder may be enlarged. Histological changes include cellular accumulation of lipids, fibrosis and extensive bile duct proliferation.

Swine: Feed containing 0.4 ppm or greater of AFB_1 fed from weaning to market weight can adversely affect the health of pigs. Among the midest affects are decreased feed efficiency and poor rate of gain. More severe effects include acute hepatitis, systemic hemorrhage and nephrosis. The extent of pathological abnormality observed in the liver and kidney was closely related to the AFB_1 level in the diet. In a swine reproduction experiment, no adverse effects were detected in piglet produced from sows fed 450 ppm aflatoxin. Moreover, piglets are more sensitive than older pigs. However, stunted growth has been observed

278

in piglet that nursed on sows fed contaminated feed since AFM_1, a toxic metabolite of AFB_1 is transferred into milk. Clear damage to liver, changes in blood and loss of appetite were observed in many pigs with 2 or 4 mg aflatoxin per day per animal.

Poultry: Avian species are quite variable insensitivity to chronic aflatoxicosis. Turkey, poultry and ducklings are the most sensitive, i.e. a dietary level of 0.25 ppm impair their growth. A level of 0.5 ppm in chickens is required to reduce growth rate and a level of 1.25 ppm or more in chicks diet resulted in increased liver lipids. A level of 2.5 ppm and above reduced the final weight of chicks significantly. Dietary concentrations of aflatoxin greater than 2 ppm can significantly diminish egg production in layers and production decreased to 50% with 10 ppm and 0% at 20 ppm. Chicken were protected again at the growth inhibiting effects of 5 ppm dietary aflatoxin when the protein in the diet was increased from 20 per cent to 30 per cent. Rickets were observed in broiler chicks fed aflatoxin containing diet and showing that aflatoxins impair the availability of bile salts in the gut, resulting in decreased absorption of fat soluble vitamins. Decreased bone strength in broilers fed aflatoxins was attributed to inadequate mineralization of bone.

Ruminants: In chronic intoxication the growing calves displayed loss of appetite and reduced growth rate while milk yield was reduced in cows. This resulted in wider feed: gain ratio. However, there was no loss of appetite. Calves are more sensitive than adult cattle. A dose level of about 0.2 mg/kg body causes reduced rate of gain and impaired blood coagulation in calves. Early metabolic indications of aflatoxicosis in calves are poor feed utilization and a rapid rise in serum alkaline phosphatase (APT) activity. Feeding of aflatoxin contaiminated cotton seed meal to young beef cattle showed reduction in growth rate and feed efficiency and gross evidence of liver damage at 0.7 and 1.0 ppm levels while no abnormalities were seen with 0.1 and 0.30 ppm levels. Cows fed daily doses of 13 mg aflatoxin either as pure B_1 or as crude mixture for 7 days showed fluctuation in feed intake and milk production.

There was a significant decrease in milk production of cows receiving crude mixture. Antireproductive effects of aflatoxins in ruminants include decreased fertility in sheep and abortion and birth of underweight calves in cattle.

Food adulterants: Food adulterants are generally mixed along with the concentrate mixture, especially when it is mash or pellet form. Individual ingredients are sometimes also found adulterated with various types od adulterants, which are not only poor in nutritive value but are also harmful to the animals. The costly feeds are generally adulterated. The fish meal is adulterated with sand, urea and salt. The grains are adulterated with water. Several adulterants are added in various bulks like rice husk, saw dust, ground nut shells, brick powder and small pieces of stones. The quality control of feed is regulated by the legislation laid down by the Bureau of Indian Standards (BIS), New Delhi. The adulterants, which are commonly mixed with foodre:

1. Sweet potato, potato and hydrogenated vegetable oils (margarine, vanaspati etc.) mixed with ghee.

2. Water and starch are mixed with milk and milk products.

3. Argimone oil mixed with mustard oil.

4. Coloured saw dust mixed with turmeric powder and tea leaves.

5. Foils of aluminium used in place of silver foil to wrap betel and sweets.

6. Besan of khesari (*Lathyrus odoratus*) mixed the besan of gram and others.

7. Sacchrin in sweets.

The adulterants may be harmless or harmful, which may cause bad effect on health. So the laboratory must be equipped with the facilities to detect the presence of adulterants in feed.

Q.1. Fill in the blanks

1. — — — — — — — —and — — — — — — are the alkaloids which are toxic to animals.

2. Hydrolysis of cyanogens produce — — — — which is a potent toxin.

3. — — — — —cyanogen is found in sudan grass.

4. Cyanide is converted into thiocyanate by enzyme — — — — — —.

5. Glucosinolates inhibit the function of — — — — — — — — gland.

6. Glucosinolates are hydrolysed by enzyme — — — — — — — —.

7. Glucosinolates toxicity produced symptoms like — — — — — — — — —.

8. Sweet clovers (*Melilotus albus*) contain a toxic glycoside known as — — —.

9. The toxicity symptoms of sweet clover poisoning are — — — — — — — —;

10. The sweet clover poisoning can be treated by injection of vitamin — — — —.

11. Saponins are glycosides found in plants like — — — — — — and — — — — — — —.

12. Trypsin inhibitors are found in plants like — — — — — — — and — — — — — — —.

13. — — — — — —treatment destroys the trypsin inhibitors.

14. Hemagglutinins cause the — — — — — — of red blood cells.

15. The toxic amino acid mimosine is found in plants — — — — — —.

16. Lathyrism is a crimpling disease produced by comsumption of — — — — seeds.

17. — — — — — —and— — — — — — crops are rich in oxalate content.

18. — — — — — — —percipitate calcium in gastrointestinal tract as calcium oxalate.

19. Phytic acid is found in plants like — — — — — — — — and — — — — — —.

20.   – – – – – – – – – depresses the utilization of many minerals specially phosphorus.

21.   – – – – – – – – – –and – – – – – – – – are the phenol derivatives which are present in many plants as toxic substances.

22.   The toxic substance present in cotton seed is – – – – – – – – – –.

23.   Tannin a toxic substance found in – – – – – – – and – – – – – – – –.

24.   ·Tannins reduce the availability of – – – – – – – by forming complex with it.

25.   – – – –, – – – – – –, – – – – – – and – – – – are the four major toxins produced by fungi.

26.   The most potent mycotoxin is – – – – – – – – –.

27.   – – – – – – –and – – – – – – – are the fungal species producing aflatoxins.

28.   The quality control of feed is regulated by the legislation laid down by the – –·- – – – – – – – – – – – – – – –.

29.   When low levels of toxin are ingested over a prolonged period results into – – – – – – – –.

30.   – – – – – – – – and – – – – – – – – are highly sensitive to aflatoxins where as – – – – -   – –and – – – – – – – – – – are less sensitive.

Q.2. Explain the following:

1.·   Define the toxin substance. How the naturally occuring toxic substances are classified?

2.   Explain the naturally occuring alkaloids and Glycosides in plants which are toxic to animals.

3.   Mention the various toxic substances which influence the protein utilization by animals.

4.   Write a note on metal binding substance and inorganic toxicants.

5.   Effect of mycotoxins in animal production.

6.   Gossypol and Tannin as harmful natural constituents of plants.

MODEL TEST PAPER- I

PART A: Objective type   MM: 40

Course No. ANN- 211 (*Principles of Animal Nutrition including avian*)

A. Fill in the blanks

1. A French chemist – – – – – – is called as father of nutrition.

2. The water which is produced in the body due to anabolic or catabolic processes is called as ....

3. The structural substance in plant is .... where as reserve material is starch.

4. Polyneuritis in birds is caused due to deficiency of ....

5. .... is the immediate source of energy in animal body.

6. Goose stepping gait appear in pig due to deficiency of..............

7. The precursor of niacin is ....

8. Proximate analysis of feed was devised by the scientists of Weende experiment.......................

9. For the absorption of vitamin B_{12} a glycoprotein is required known as.............

10. . ... a vitamin which is constituent of lecithin.

B. Write T for true and F for false against each statement

1. Gluconeogenesis is a process of glycogen synthesis from glucose.

2. When 7-dehydrocholesterol is exposed to U.V. rays, it is converted to cholecalciferol.

3. Arachidonic acid is an essential fatty acid required for the synthesis of prostaglandin.

4. Niacin is vitamin of B- complex group is function as two co- enzyme known as NAD and FAD.

5. In ruminants, vitamin B$_{12}$ is not a dietary essential but cobalt is a dietary essential where as in non ruminants, vitamin B$_{12}$ is a dietary essential but cobalt is not a dietary essential.

C. Choose the most appropriate option

1. Swollen hock syndrome in chicks due to deficiency of-
    a. Mn b. Zn c. Ca d. Fe
2. Anaemia is due to deficiency of-
    a. Cu b. Co c. Fe d. Zn
3. The term polyunsaturated fatty acid is applied to those unsaturated fatty acid which have-
    a. More than one double bond
    b. More than two double bond
    c. More than three double bond
    d. More than four double bond
4. Sulpher containing vitamin is-
    a. Choline & Biotin   b. Biotin & thiamin
    c. Biotin & Pyridoxine   d. Choline & thiamin
5. Steely wool in sheep is due to deficiency of-
    a. Cu b. Se c. Zn d. Mn

Course No. ANN- 212 (*Evaluation of feed stuffs and feed technology*)

A. Fill in the blanks

1. One gram methane contains .... K cal gross energy.
2. Metabolizable energy minus net energy is equal to ....
3. .... is best forage crop for hay making.
4. ......:......... is a toxic factor present in linseed.
5. Starch equivalent system was established by a German scientist known as ....
6. Neutral detergent fiber consists of acid detergent fiber and ....

7. The feeding stuffs containing less than 18 percent crude fiber but more than 20percent crude protein are commonly referred as ....

8. The factor 6.25 is multiplied with nitrogen percent to get the protein content of the feeds as on average all the feed proteins contain .... percent nitrogen .

9. The true biological value was calculated for the first time by .... modifying the procedure originated by Thomas for biological value.

10. By feeding poor quality roughages there is increase in heat increment because of the increase in production of .... in the rumen.

B. Write T for true and F for false against each statement

1. Feed material can be stored safely for longer duration when the moisture content is less than 12%.

2. Lignin is a carbohydrate but not digested by non ruminants as they lack enzyme for its digestion.

3. Gossypol which is a toxic substance present in cotton seed.

4. Maize fodder is the best crop for hay making because it is rich in soluble carbohydrates.

5. Basal feeds are those feeds which contain less than 20 percent crude protein but more than 18 percent crude fiber.

C. Choose the most appropriate option

1. Dry matter content of the crop for silage making showed be-

   a. 28 % b. 35% c. 42% d. 49%

2. One kilogram of TDN is equivalent to-

   a. 3.2Mcal ME b. 3.4Mca ME c. 3.6Mcal ME d. 3.8Mcal ME

3. The best system for expressing the energy value of feeds is-

   A. Gross energy   B. Metabolizable energy

   C. Total digestible nutrients   D.Net energy

4. Subabool contains a toxic factor known as-
   A. Mimosin B. Salanine
   C. Nimbine D. None of the above
5. In the milk factor used for converting the nitrogen content into protein is-
   a. 6.25 b. 6.38 c. 5.75 d. 5.38

PART B: Subjective type   MM: 60

Course No. ANN- 211 (*Principles of Animal Nutrition including avian*)

Attempt all questions from each part.

Q. 1. Write short notes on:

a. By pass protein

b.Ca and P absorption

c. Vit. K and blood coagulation

d. Metabolic water

Q. 2. Write in detail on the following:

(a). discuss the importance of Fe and Cu in animal nutrition. what is the relation between these two minerals?

(b).   microbial protein

Q. 3. Discuss the following in detail:

(a). Milk fever and pica

(b). Utilization of NPN compounds in ruminants

OR

Discuss in detail the metabolism of carbohydrates in ruminants and also discuss the factors affecting volatile fatty acid absorption.

Course No. ANN- 212 (*Evaluation of feed stuffs and feed technology*)

1. Write short notes on the following:

a. physiological fuel value

b. Scandinavian feed unit system

c. Animal protein supplements

d. Chemical score

2.   Write in detail on the following:

(a). Give procedure for urea ammoniation of poor quality roughages. Also give precaution while feeding the treated material (b). Heat production measurement in animals and its limitations.

3.   Discuss the following:

   (a). Can we prepare silage from leguminous crops? If yes how? If not why?

   (b). What is the best biological method for expressing feed protein quality for poultry?

OR

Name various natural antinutritional substances present in feedstuffs. Discuss HCN toxicity in detail.

MODEL TEST PAPER- II

PART A: Objective type   **MM: 40**

Course No. ANN- 211 (*Principles of Animal Nutrition including avian*)

A. True or false

1. In nylon bag technique, nylon bags are incubated in the rumen for longer time for concentrates as compare to roughages.

2. If particle size of feed is too small the digestibility of feed decreases.

3. The energy requirement in sheep grazing on pasture is higher than under stall feeding.

4. The main anti nutritional factor present in tree leaves is oxalic acid.

5. Restriction of feed in poultry feeding is helpful in achieving eggs of larger size.

B. Fill in the blanks

1. Piglets require supplementation of mineral known as ....as it is deficient in milk.

2. Low blood calcium in high milk producing cows leads to.................

3. Mahua seed cake is not palatable to the animals as it contains anti nutritional substance known as ....

4. Perosis in chicks occur due to the deficiency of mineral known as................

5. Yellow maize contains a precursor of vitamin known as.........

6. Enlargement of liver and kidneys and scouring occurs in swine on excess consumption of...............

7. Calves should be fed........... % milk of their body weight.

8. Feed additive known as................. is used as antioxidant in the feed.

9. Calorie protein ratio in broiler starter feed is .... than broiler finisher feed.

10. Energy value of feeds expressed as Starch equivalent was given by...............

C. Encircle the correct answer from the following-

1. Theoretically respiratory quotient value during fasting is-
   a. 0.7 b. 0.8 c. 0.9 d. 1.0

2. Digestibility of roughage feed is determined by incubating nylon bags in rumen for-
   a. 60 hrs b. 72 hrs c. 48 hrs. d. 36 hrs.

3. Following amount of concentrate mixture, on an average basis, should be given to cattle (producing 10 liters of milk) for the production of each kg of milk-
   a. 100 g. b. 200 g. c. 350 g. d. 500 g.

4. Natural indicator (marker) used for the determination of digestibility of feed in animal is-
   a. polyethylene glycol b. carmine c. chromic oxide d. lignin

5. Which of the following is a leguminous fodder-
   a. Lucerne b. Mustard c. Sorghum d. Maize

Course No. ANN- 212 (*Evaluation of feed stuffs and feed technology*)

A. True or false

i. A slight alkaline pH in rumen increases the rate of absorption of VFA.

ii. Zinc prevents or cures parakeratosis in poultry.

iii. Probiotic are living organism.

iv. Amino acid is NPN compound.

v. Collagen being protein contain cystine and cystein

B. Fill in the blanks.

1. .... moles of ATP are produced from the oxidation of one mole of butyric acid.

2. The number of amino acid essential for poultry is ....

3. The quality of metabolic faecal nitrogen in ruminants is .... mg/100g DMI.

4. .... an essential fatty acid is used for the synthesis of other essential fatty acid.

5. Copper is integral part of enzyme ....

6. Metabolic water produced per gram of fat is........

7. Pellagra is disease caused by deficiency of ....

8. The major gases produced due to fermentation of carbohydrates are CO_2 and ....

9. Conversion of propionate to glucose requires vitamin Biotin and ....

10. The biological value of microbial protein is........percent.

C. Encircle the correct answer from the following—

1. The recommended level of adding urea in concentrate mixture —

   a. 1%   b. 2%

   c. 3%   d. 4%

2. The factor for calculating protein in milk from nitrogen is —

   a. 6.25   b. 6.38

   c. 5.71   d. 5.75

3. Glutathione peroxidase is associated with—

   a. Vitamin-E b. Selenium

   c. Cobalt   d. Molybdenum

4. Pepsin breaks the peptide chain where amino acid —

   a. Lysine   b. Arginine

   c. Glycine   d. Tyrosine

5. Brown fat is found in

   a. Lamb   b. Calf

   c. Dog   d. Chicken

PART B: Subjective type   MM: 60

Course No. ANN- 211 (*Principles of Animal Nutrition including avian*)

Attempt all questions from each part.

1. Discuss the digestion, absorption and metabolism of carbohydrates in sheep.

2. Write short notes on the following:

   a. Interrelationship between amino acids and vitamins.

   b. Interrelationship between vitamin A and night blindness.

   c. Mucosal block theory for iron absorption.

   d. Essential amino acids for ruminants and non ruminants.

   e. Feed additives.

3. (a). Write the general functions of minerals in the body.

   (b). Discuss how non protein nitrogenous compounds are utilize in bullocks.

Course No. ANN- 212 (*Evaluation of feed stuffs and feed technology*)

Q. 1. (a). Give the out line of classification of feeds and fodder.

   (b). What do you mean by inferior quality roughages? How will you improve the nutritive value of paddy straw in your locality?

Q. 2. Define and explain the following terms:

   a. Starch equivalent

   b. Metabolic water

   c. Heat increment

   d. Nutritive ratio

   e. Essential amino acid

   f. Biological value

   g. Animal Nutrition

h. Protein efficiency ratio

i. Milestones of animal nutrition

j. Feed technology

Q. 3. What do you mean by antinutritional factor? Discuss the different antinutritional substances that depress the protein utilization in animals.

MODEL TEST PAPER- III

PART A: Objective type   **MM: 40**

Course No. ANN- 211 (*Principles of Animal Nutrition including avian*)

A. Write true or false.

1. Per unit body weight, the water requirement in birds is less than mammals.

2. In animals' body, structural material is protein whereas reserve material is fat.

3. Amino peptidase act on the peptide bond adjacent to the free amino group of simple peptides whereas, dipeptidase splits the dipeptides to free amino acids.

4. The immunoglobulins present in colostrums are absorbed in new born mammals by a process known as pinocytosis.

5. The deficiency of vitamin B_1 (thiamin) in birds causes curled-toe paralysis.

6. Star grazing is a symptom of pantothenic acid deficiency in pigs.

7. High phosphorus intake along with calcium leads to formation of mineral deposit in bladder of sheep.

8. Tryptophan serves as precursor of melanin pigment.

B. Fill in the blanks.

1. The trypsinogen is converted into trypsin by the action of an enzyme liberated from duodenal mucosa known as ....

2. The absorption of calcium is regulated by an intermediate metabolite of vitamin D known as ....

3. In cellulose the linkage between glucose molecule is.............................

4. Copper plays an important role in production of crimp in wool. The deficiency of copper causes break in wool fiber and the condition is commonly known as.............

5. The detergent system of partitioning fiber was evolved by ....

6. The net ATP produced from the oxidation of propionic acid in sheep is ....

7. ....is a mineral required in blood coagulation as it helps   in conversion of prothrombin into thrombin.

8. .... is a constituent of respiratory enzyme, carbonic anhydrase.

C. Choose the most appropriate answer.

1. Muscular dystrophy in chicks is due to deficiency of which enzyme?

    a.   cholecalciferol b. α- tocopherol c. retinol d. none of the above

2. Ketosis in high yielding cow can be prevented by giving

    a.   fat rich diet   b. protein rich diet

    c.   mineral rich diet   d. soluble carbohydrate rich diet.

3. Which of the following vitamin is required during conversion of Tryptophan into niacin?

    a. thiamin b. riboflavin c. pyridoxine d. biotin

4. One molecule ATP yields energy —-

    a. 7.3 Kcal b. 8.3 Kcal c. 12.6 Kcal d. 14.6 Kcal

Course No. ANN- 212 (*Evaluation of feed stuffs and feed technology*)

Write true or false

1. Chaffing of green forage increases the surface area for enzymatic digestion in rumen.

2. Paddy straw contains a toxic substance known as mimosine.

3. Heat increment from feeding of roughage is less than from feeding of concentrates.

4. The measure of protein quality in which percent of protein intake which is actually utilized is referred to as biological value.

5. One gram methane produced in rumen causes loss of 13.34 Kcal gross energy.

6. The feed material can be stored safely when moisture content of it is less than 12 percent.

7. For hay making, the forage crops having thick stem are generally preferred.

8. Bone meal is a source of both calcium and phosphorus.

B. Fill in the blanks.

1. ....% of digestible energy is Metabolizable energy in ruminants.

2. .... serves as hydrogen sink in the rumen.

3. .... are those feeding stuff which contain less than 18% crude fiber and more than 55% TDN on air dry basis.

4. The physiological value of carbohydrate is.................

5. In oat hay poisoning the blood haemoglobin is converted into irreversible methemoglobin due to presence of toxic substance known as ....

6. The dry matter content of forage crop at the time of ensiling should be .... %.

7. The nutritive ratio in wheat / paddy straw is ....

8. The factor 6.25 is multiplied with nitrogen content in the feed to obtain protein content because on an average protein contains .... % nitrogen.

C. Choose the most appropriate answer.

1. The pH value of good silage range from-

    a. 3.7 to 4.2 b. 4.3 to 4.8 c. 4.9 to 5.4 d. 5.5 to 6.0

2. Which of the following feed ingredients is not a protein supplement?

    a. groundnut cake b. mustard cake c. soyabean meal d. maize grain

3. Scandinavian food unit system is based on the net energy value of one kg of -
   a. oats b. barley c. maize d. wheat
4. Which of the following is also known as king of fodder crop-
   a. Maize b. Sorghum c. Berseem d. Lucerne

PART B: Subjective type **MM: 60**

Course No. ANN- 211 (*Principles of Animal Nutrition including avian*)

Attempt any three questions from each part.

Q.1. Write short note on the following (any five)

a.   Hemi cellulose

b.   Phospholipids

c.   Factors affecting crude fibre digestion

d.   Composition of animal body

e.   Chemical properties of fats

f.   Enzootic ataxia

Q.2. Enlist the various proximate principles of feed stuff. Describe briefly the nutritional importance of each proximate principle.

Q.3. Describe in detail the digestion and absorption of protein in monogastric animals.

Q.4. What do you mean by metabolic water? Write the properties and functions of water in animal body.

Course No. ANN- 212 (*Evaluation of feed stuffs and feed technology*)

1.   What are the various system for expressing the energy value of feed? Discuss all the system with their merits and demerits.

2.   Enlist the various antinutritional factors present in livestock feed/fodder and discuss about two of these antinutritional factors with the measure to ameliorate them.

3.   Explain with reason/ answer the following in two or three lines:

a.   For determination of biological value of a protein, enough carbohydrate and fats should be supplemented in diet.

b.   The digestibility of cellulose in feeds gets reduced when molasses is added to a feed.

c.   The digestibility coefficient of ash is generally not determined and digestible ash is not considered while calculating the TDN value of feed.

d.   Fine grinding of low grade roughage reduces the dry matter digestibility.

e.   Bone meal should be sterilized before using in the ration of animals.

4.   Describe the carbon nitrogen balance method for measuring heat production in animals.

MODEL TEST PAPER- IV

PART A: Objective type   **MM: 40**

Course No. ANN- 211 (*Principles of Animal Nutrition including avian*)

A: Fill the blanks with appropriate words. No cutting and overwriting are allowed.

1. The non-protein group in conjugated protein is called — — — — — — — — — — — — — — — .

2. The process of separation of nitrogen from an amino acid in the form of ammonia is called — — — — — — — — — — — — — — — .

3. A net gain of — — — — — — — — — — — — — — moles of ATP is produced by 1 mole palmitic acid metabolism.

4. The absorption of galactose is — — — — — — — — — — than glucose at intestinal level.

5. The separation of acetyl CoA from fatty acids yields — — — — — — — moles of ATP.

6.   Milking animals require — — — — — — — — — — — — — — kg water per kg milk produced.

B: Encircle T for True and F for False against in each statement accordingly:

(i)   Age of maturity and lignin content of feed increases digestibility in cattle.   T/ F

(ii)   Conjugated proteins are composed of simple protein combined with some non- protein substances. T/ F

(iii) Cellulose is equally digested by sheep and horse.   T/ F

(iv) True digestibility is always higher than apparent digestibility of a feed.   T/F

C: Match the column A with column B as space provided against the words of column A:

Column A   Write answer   Column B

(a) Milk fever   1. Blood clotting

(b) Cellulose and   2. Insoluble carbohydrate
     hemicellulose

(c) Vitamin B   3. Decreased digestibility of feed

(d) Vitamin K   4. Lamb and kid

(e) Roughage   5. Calcium

(f) Vitamin E   6. Gas accumulation in rumen

(g) Lignin content   7. Not required in ruminants

(h) Finisher ration   8. Phosphorous

(i) Bloat   9. Anti sterility factor

(j) Pica   10. More than 65% TDN

Course No. ANN- 212 (*Evaluation of feed stuffs and feed technology*)

A: Fill the blanks with appropriate words. No cutting and overwriting are allowed.

1. One kg of TDN =.......... M cal of ME.

2. One gram of protein retained in the body is equivalent to .... k cal.

3. Two non-leguminous forage crops of rabi season are .... and oat.

4. Net protein value=............ × CP.

5. The minimum requirement for efficient lignocellulose break down of roughages fed as a sole diet is.............

6. Most of the cereals are deficient in vitamin......

7. Crops rich in ....:. are most suitable for silage making.

8. In ammonia treatment of roughages, ammonia is added as.........../100 kg.

9. Beet molasses contain..........% CP.

10. The heat increment includes heat of fermentation and
    ....

B: Encircle T for True and F for False against in each statement accordingly:

1. Most of the feeds used in the ruminants ration contain 4.4-4.5 Mcal /g DM.
2. Poor quality feeds are underestimated for their energy content by the TDN system.
3. Biological value of protein is maximum at maintenance level.
4. Determination of TDN does not require a digestion trial but chemical analysis of feeds and faeces requires.
5. Bound gossypol is less toxic than free gossypol.

C. Tick (√) the correct option—

1. CP content (%) of wheat straw is-
   a. 1.5 b. 1.2 c. 6.5 d. 3.5
2. To calculate SE one part of digestible fat from wheat straw is multiplied by-factor —
   a. 2.41 b. 2.12 c. 1.71 d. 1.91
3. CO_2 produced (liter) by each gram of protein oxidized is-
   a. 0.77 b. 0.96 c. 0.85 d. 0.70
4. The R.Q. of protein is —
   a. 0.7 b. 0.9 c. 1.0 d. none of the above
5. Mimosin a toxic substance present in-
   a. Lucerne leaf meal
   b. Linseed meal
   c. Rapeseed meal
   d. Subabool meal

PART B: Subjective type   MM: 60

Course No. ANN- 211 (*Principles of Animal Nutrition including avian*)

Attempt any three questions from each part and each question carry equal marks.

Q.1. Differentiate between the following

   a. Maltose and Cellobiose.

   b. Balanced ration and Purified diet.

   c. Fibrous protein and Globular protein.

   d. Grass staggers and Blind staggers.

   e. Basal metabolism and Fasting metabolism.

   f. Lecithin and Cephalin.

   g. Pernicious anaemia and Megaloblastic anaemia.

   h. Vitamin D_2 and Vitamin D_3.

   i. Crude protein and True protein.

   j. Roughage and Concentrate.

Q.2. Define the following term in two or three line.

   a. Antioxidant.

   b. Carbohydrate.

   c. Nutrient.

   d. Rancidity in fat.

   e. Feed additives.

   f. Feed conversion efficiency.

   g. Stover.

   h. Provitamines.

   i. Saponification number.

   j. Basal feeds.

Q.3. Write short notes on the following (any five).

   a. Non-protein nitrogen utilization in cattle.

   b. Swine parakeratosis.

   c. β-oxidation

d. Function of fats.

e. Glycolytic cycle.

f. Exudative diathesis.

Q.4. (a) Classify minerals and discuss the general function of mineral in animal body.

(b) Describe the microbial digestion and absorption of carbohydrates in goat.

Course No. ANN- 212 (*Evaluation of feed stuffs and feed technology*)

Q.1. Define the following term in two or three line.

a) Objective of feed processing.

b) Feed Technology.

c) Respiratory quotient.

d) Protein efficiency ratio.

e) Ration and diet.

f) Soaking.

g) Silage

h) Alkali treatment of straw

i) Micronization

j) Heat increment

Q.2. Differentiate between the following.

a) Total digestible nutrient and Metabolizable energy

b) Silage and Wastelage

c) Nutritive ratio and Calorie : protein ratio

d) Starch equivalent and Net energy

e) Net protein utilization and Net protein value

f) Digestible crude protein and Protein equivalent

g) Direct calorimetry and Indirect calorimetry

h) Feed and Food

i) Cubbing and Pelleting

j) Stover and Kadbi

Q.3. Write short notes on any four of the following.
   a) Animal by products
   b) Feed adulterants
   c) Characteristic of good hay and silage
   d) Poor quality roughages
   e) Importance of green forage

Q.4. What are cakes? Discuss ghani, expeller and solvent extracted cakes with suitable examples.

MODEL TEST PAPER- V

PART A: Objective type   **MM: 40**

Course No. ANN- 211 (*Principles of Animal Nutrition including avian*)

Attempt all questions and each question carries 0.5 marks.
Q. 1. Tick mark (√) the most suitable choice from the answer given below.

(1). Protein molecules are joined together through-

(a) H_2 bonding (b) Covalent bond (c) Peptide bond (d) none

(2). The number of total essential amino acids for poultry is-

(a) 9   (b) 10   (c) 11

(d) None of the above

(3). Curled toe paralysis in poultry is deficiency symptoms of-

(a) Thiamine (b) Pantothenic acid

(c) Choline (d) Riboflavin

(4). Osteomalacia is deficiency symptoms of -

(a) Calcium   (b) Phosphorous

(c) Vitamin D   (d) All of the above

(5). Vitamin K was identified by the scientist-

(a) Mc Collum   (b) Dam   (c) Evans   (d) Eijkman

(6). Which of the following fatty acids is responsible for milk fat synthesis in cow?

(a) Acetic acid   (b) Propionic acid

(c) Butyric acid   (d) Valine

(7). Lysine content of the ration increases by mixing the following ingredients-

(a) Bone meal (b) Mustard cake (c) Groundnut cake (d) Soybean meal

(8). A condition known as "Teartness" is due to toxicity of-
(a) Chromiun   (b) Cobalt
(c) Selenium   (d) Molybdenum

(9). In equal concentration which of the following monosaccharide is absorbed at the fastest rate from the intestine?
(a) Galactose   (b) Glucose
(c) Fructose   (d) Mannose

(10). Number of net ATP formed per mole of butyric acid oxidized are-
(a) 2   (b) 38   (c) 25   (d) 8

Q. 2. Fill in the blanks with most suitable word-

1. In blood clotting process a mineral known as — — — — play an important role.

2. A nutrient known as — — — — — — increases in plants with advancing maturity.

3. Pica in cattle occurs due to deficiency of mineral called as — — — — — — —.

4. Stiff lamb disease is caused by — — — — — — — — — — — —.

5. Fatty acids are metabolized by — — — — — — — — — — — — — — —.

6. The pancreatic enzymes viz. — — — — — — — and — — — — — — — — — attack the partial breakdown product of protein in the duodenum.

7. One IU of vitamin D is equal to — — — — — — — — — — — —.

8. Chemical name of vitamin K is — — — — — — — — — — — — —.

9. Niacine is prosthetic group in co-enzymes namely — — — — — — and — — — — —.

10. Acetyl number is mg of — — — — — required to combined with acetic acid liberated by saponification of one gram of acetylated fat.

Q. 3. State whether following statements are TRUE/ FALSE-

1. Linolenic acid is the most essential fatty acid for non ruminants.
2. Lignin is present in secondary cell wall of plant cell in high quantity.
3. Vegetable oils are poor source of vitamin E and essential fatty acids.
4. The production of propionic acid decreases if the proportion of concentrate is increased in the diet of ruminants.
5. Curled toe paralysis in chicks is caused due to deficiency of riboflavin.
6. Peat scour is caused by deficiency of folacin.
7. Protein is considered as building block material of the body.
8. During fasting, blood glucose level increases in animals.
9. Omasum, a part of stomach is present in camel and absent in goat.
10. Concentrates are poor quality protein source for small ruminants feeding.

Q. 4. Match the following

( ) i) Calcium	a) Rickets
( ) ii) Selenium	b) Blind staggers
( ) iii) Manganese	c) Vitamin B$_{12}$
( ) iv) Cobalt	d) Slipped tendon/ perosis
( ) v) Zinc	e) Milk fever
( ) vi) Choline	f) Exudative diathesis
( ) vii) Vitamin D	g) Black tongue
( ) viii) Vitamin A	h) Parakeratosis
( ) xi) Vitamin K	i) Blood clotting
( ) x) Niacin	j) Night blindness

Course No. ANN- 212 (*Evaluation of feed stuffs and feed technology*)

Q. 1. Tick mark (Ö) the most suitable choices from the answer given below.

1. Thin stem crops are conserved as-
   (a) Hay   (b) Silage
   (c) Silo   (d) None of the above

2. Crops selected for ensiling process should have dry matter-
   (a) 20-30%   (b) 30-35%
   (c) 35-45%   (d) None of the above

3. Urea is added in silage making to improve the-
   (a) CO_2 content   (b) N_2 content
   (c) S_2 content   (d) None of the above

4. Aflatoxin is-
   (a) Bacterial toxin   (b) Viral toxin
   (c) Fungal toxin   (d) Protozoal toxin

5. Mustard cake contains-
   (a) 5% CP   (b) 7% CP
   (c) 11% CP   (d) None of these

6. DCP is a measure that has been widely used to evaluate the protein for-
   (a) Non-ruminant   (b) Ruminant
   (c) Both of these   (d) None of the above

7. In general, young leaves contain oxalic acid than mature leaves in-
   (a) Higher amount   (b) Lower amount
   (c) Medium amount   (d) None

8. Ochratoxins are-
   (a) Premix   (b) Additives
   (c) Mycotoxins   (d) None of these

9. Gross energy of fat is-
   (a) 4.090 Kcal/g (b) 9.400 Kcal/g
   (c) 4.900 Kcal/g (d) None of these

10. Groundnut cake contains-
    (a) 10% CP   (b) 13% CP
    (c) 5% CP   (d) None of these

Q. 2. Fill in the blanks with most suitable word-

1. Food proteins contain — — — — — — — — — — — — percent N_2.

2. Molasses should be added @ — — — — — — —percent for
   silage making.

3. For good quality silage making plant material should be
   stored at a moisture content of — — — — — — — — — —
   percent.

4. Productive type of roughages contain more than — — — —
   —percent DCP.

5. Outer covering of grains and grams is called — — — — — —
   — — — —.

6. 1 kg TDN = — — — — — — — — — — Mcal DE.

7. Feed mixers are of two types — — — — — — — and — — —
   — — — — — — — —.

8. Concentrate feeds are classified into — — — — — — — — —
   — — groups.

9. In ensiling process, due to fermentation, organic acids
   which are produced are — — — — — — —, — — — — — — —
   — — — — and — — — — — — — — — — — — —.

10. Sweet clover disease is due to — — — — — — — — — — com-
    pound.

Q. 3. State whether following statements are TRUE/ FALSE-

1. Meals contain higher fat than cake.

2. Straw contains zero percent DCP.

3. Energy of heat increment is wasted when the temperature
   of environment is below the critical level.

4. Feeds richer in protein have narrow nutritive value.
5. Urea and biurate is a NPN compound.
6. Selective feeding by livestock will be minimized by grinding or pelleting.
7. Crops with thick stem are conserved in the form of hay.
8. Crops rich in soluble sugars are not suitable for ensiling.
9. Oxalic acid is not an antinutritional factor.
10. Aflatoxin is a mycotoxin.

Q. 4. Match the following

( ) i) Aflatoxin   a) Pelleting
( ) ii) Saponin   b) Inositol
( ) iii) Protein   c) Roasting
( ) iv) Cyanogen   d) Stean rolling
( ) v) Gossypol   e) Antinutritional factor
( ) vi) Phytic acid   f) Mycotoxin
( ) vii) Selective feeding   g) 16% N_2
( ) viii) Dry processing method   h) > 18% crufe fibre
( ) xi) Wet processing method   i) Cyanide
( ) x) Roughage   j) Cotton seed

PART B: Subjective type　　　　**MM: 60**

Course No. ANN- 211 (*Principles of Animal Nutrition including avian*)

Attempt any three questions from each part.

Q.1. Name the various macro elements. Discuss the role of calcium and phosphorus in the feeding of livestock.

Q.2. Discuss the crude fiber metabolism in ruminants.

Q.3. What are proteins? Give the detail classification of proteins with suitable examples.

Q.4. Name various proximate principles of feed. Discuss their importance in feeding in livestock.

Q.5. What is vitamin A? Discuss its role in feeding of livestock and poultry.

Course No. ANN- 212 (*Evaluation of feed stuffs and feed technology*)

1. Give the detailed classification of feeding stuffs commonly fed to livestock and poultry with suitable example.

2. Name the various techniques used for improving the nutritive value of inferior quality roughages. Discuss the most commonly used techniques.

3. Define TDN. How it differs from starch equivalent. Discuss the merits and demerits of TDN system.

4. What is biological value of protein? Discuss in detail the Thomas-Mitchal method used for working out it.

5. Define silage, How would you prepare a good quality silage of green jowar fodder?

Livestock population in million (FAO, 2003)

Animal species	India	World	Global Population in India (%)
Cattle	226.1	1371.1	16.49
Buffalo	96.9	170.7	56.77
Sheep	59.0	1024.0	5.76
Goat	124.5	767.9	16.21
Swine	18.5	956.0	1.93
Horse	0.8	55.5	1.44
Mule	0.3	12.8	2.34
Ass	0.8	40.3	1.99
Camel	0.9	19.1	4.71
Total	527.8	4417.4	11.95

Reference Books of General Animal Nutrition Used in India

1. Banerjee G.C. (1999). A Text Book of Animal husbandry, 8th edition, Oxford & IBH Publishing Co. Pvt. Ltd., Calcutta.

2. Banerjee G.C. (1999). Feeds and Principles of Animal Nutrition, 2nd edition, reprint 1999, Oxford & IBH Publishing Co. Pvt. Ltd., Calcutta.

3. Crampton E. W. and Harris L.E. (1968). Applied Animal Nutrition, 2nd edition.

4. E.J. Underwood (1977). Trace Elements in Human and Animal Nutrition, 4th edition, 5th edition by Walter Mertz 1987, CABI Publishing, New York, USA.

5. Handbook of Animal Husbandry (2003). ICAR, New Delhi.

6. Hungate R.E. (1966). The Rumen and its Microbes, 1st edition.

7. Lassiter J.W. and Edwards H.M., Jr.(1982). Animal Nutrition, 1st edition.

8. Maynard L.A., Loosli J.K., Hintz H.F. and Warner R.G. (1979). Animal Nutrition, 7th edition, Tata McGraw-Hill Publishing Co. Ltd, New Delhi.

9. Mc Donald P., Edwards R.A., Greenhalgh J.F.D and Morgan, C.A. (2004). Animal Nutrition, 6th edition, Tata McGraw-Hill Publishing Co. Ltd, New Delhi.

10. Mc Dowell L.R. (1989). Vitamin in Animal Nutrition (Comparative Aspects to Human Nutrition), 1st edition, Academic Press California, USA.

11. Mc Dowell L.R. (1992). Minerals in Animal and Human Nutrition, 1st edition, Academic Press California, USA.

12. Mudgal V.D., Singhal K.K. and Sharma D.D. (1995). Advanced Animal Nutrition for Developing Countries, 1st edition.

13. Mugdal V.D., Singhal K.K. and Sharma D.D. (1995). Advances in Dairy Animal Production, 1ˢᵗ edition.

14. Pandey D.N. and Bajpai Amita, (2003). Recent Trends in Animal Nutrition and Feed Technology for Livestock, Pets and Laboratory Animals, 1ˢᵗ edition, International Book Distributing Company, Lucknow.

15. Pathak N.N. (1997). Textbook of Feed Processing Technology, 1ˢᵗ edition, Vikas Publishing House, New Delhi.

16. Pathak N.N. and Jakhmola, R. (1983). Forage and Livestock Production, Vikas Publishing House, New Delhi.

17. Prasad J. (1997). Animal Husbandry and Dairy Science, 1ˢᵗ edition, Kalyani Publishers, Ludhiana.

18. Ranjhan S.K. (1991). Chemical Composition and Nutritive Value of Indian Feeds and Feeding of Farm Animals, 1ˢᵗ edition.

19. Ranjhan S.K. (1998). Nutrient Requirements of Livestock and Poultry 2ⁿᵈ revised edition, ICAR, New Delhi.

20. Ranjhan, S.K. (1990). Agro Industrial by Products and Non Conventional Feeds for Livestock Feeding, Vikas Publishing House, New Delhi.

21. Ranjhan, S.K. (1997). Animal Nutrition in the Tropics: 4ᵗʰ edition, Vikas Publishing House, New Delhi.

22. Reddy D.V. (2001). Principle of Animal Nutrition and Feed Technology, 1ˢᵗ edition, Oxford & IBH Publishing Co. Pvt. Ltd., Calcutta.

23. Sen K.C., Ray S.N. and Ranjhan S. K. (1978). Nutritive value of Indian Cattle Feeds and Feeding of Animals, 6ᵗʰ edition, ICAR, New Delhi.

24. Singhal K.K. (1992). Dictionary of Animal Nutrition and Feed Technology, 1ˢᵗ edition.

25. Swaminathan K. (1989). Principles of Nutrition and Dietetics, 2ⁿᵈ edition.

26. Underwood E.J. and Suttle N.F. (1999). The Mineral Nutrition of Livestock, 3ʳᵈ edition, CABI Publishing, New York, USA.

27. Verma, D.N. (1999). A Text Book of Livestock Production Management in Tropic, reprint 2005 Kalyani Publishers, Ludhiana.

28. Verma, D.N. (2006). A Text Book of Animal Nutrition, 2nd revised edition, Kalyani Publishers, Ludhiana.

Index